THE CLITORAL TRUTH

THE CLITORAL TRUTH
The Secret World at Your Fingertips

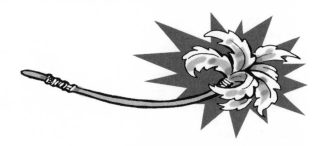

REBECCA CHALKER

ILLUSTRATIONS BY FISH

SEVEN STORIES PRESS
New York · London · Sydney · Toronto

Seven Stories Press
140 Watts Street
New York, NY 10013
http://www.sevenstories.com

In Canada: Hushion House, 36 Northline Road, Toronto, Ontario M4B 3E2

In the U.K.: Turnaround Publisher Services Ltd., Unit 3, Olympia Trading Estate, Coburg Road, Wood Green, London N22 6TZ

In Australia: Tower Books, 9/19 Rodborough Road, Frenchs Forest NSW 2086

Library of Congress Cataloging-in-Publication Data

Chalker, Rebecca.
    The clitoral truth: the world at your fingertips / Rebecca Chalker.—A Seven Stories Press first ed.
        p. cm.
ISBN 1-58322-038-0
        1. Masturbation. 2. Clitoris. 3. Women—Sexual behavior. I. Title.

HQ447.C53 2000
306.77'2—dc21

                                                        00-030790

9 8 7 6 5 4 3 2 1

College professors may order examination copies of Seven Stories Press titles for a free six-month trial period. To order, visit www.sevenstories.com/textbook, or fax on school letterhead to (212) 226-1411.

Book design by Cindy LaBreacht

Printed in the U.S.A.

CONTENTS

This book is dedicated
to the feminist activists
whose trailblazing work
helped make a new vision
of sexuality possible.

ACKNOWLEDGMENTS

First of all, eternal gratitude to my sisters and colleagues at the Federation of Feminist Women's Health Centers, past and present, for their dramatic reinterpretation of how we define the "clitoris," which began my own long and interesting journey to this book. I also thank them for their unflagging dedication to women's reproductive health, and their long and mostly unacknowledged stand on the front lines of the anti-abortion war. Sisters, salud!

Next, I'd like to thank many who helped me over the years shape this book into its final form: Lynn Rosen who did an incisive critique of an early book proposal; Shelby Lynn Brown, for her interest and help with an earlier version of this book; Mary Beth Caschetta, former editor of the SIECUS Report, who invited me to do an article, "Updating the Model of Female Sexuality" (June/July 1994), which led to my publisher Dan Simon's interest in a book on women's sexuality; Dan for his commitment to publishing socially significant work and for his extraordinary patience which allowed me to work at my own plodding pace; my editor, Kera Bolonik, for seeing the real book inside of a larger manuscript and for her sophisticated insights into the often thorny issues of sexuality; Jennifer Hengen, my agent, for believing in me and for her keen understanding of the shifting sands of the literary marketplace; my colleagues in the Lily Langtree Study Group, which explores and critiques sexuality issues—they kept me sane! I am also deeply grateful to the many women who so generously shared their personal experiences with me, as well as to the activists and sexologists who I interviewed. Special thanks to Amy Levine, librarian at the SIECUS Library for her generous assistance, and to the Lesbian Herstory Archives for making their resources available. Finally, I'd like to thank my family, which has supported me with unconditional love, even though they don't always understand what I have chosen to do.

The title, The Clitoral Truth, came to me one day while I was working on the manuscript and I knew it was perfect. Later, while reading Linda Grant's *Sexing the Millennium,* I found the phrase used as an epigram and was reminded that I had seen it in a poem by Margaret S. Chalmers in *The Spare Rib Reader,* which I bought in London in the summer of 1982.

INTRODUCTION

The women's health movement emerged from abortion reform activism in the late 1960s, becoming an important component of the second wave of feminism, and I am privileged to have been a part of it through my work at the Federation of Feminist Women's Health Centers (FFWHCs), an association of more than a dozen women's clinics based on the West Coast, with centers in Atlanta, Georgia, and Tallahassee, Florida, my hometown. The FFWHCs grew out of an abortion referral service in Los Angeles that was openly active before the *Roe v. Wade* decision was handed down in 1973. Two months after the decision, the group opened the first freestanding abortion clinic in the United States, opening others in the following five years. These clinics became part of a nationwide network of women-owned clinics and health information centers that flourished in the 1970s and 1980s. Carol Downer, founder and longtime CEO of the group, and Lorraine Rothman, founder of the Orange County FWHC in Santa Ana, California, true godmothers of the women's health movement, promoted the concept of self-empowerment and self-knowledge through the use of a personal plastic speculum, which made the vagina, previously a province solely of gynecologists, accessible to women themselves. I worked at the Tallahassee Feminist Women's Health Center, cofounded by my friend Lynn Heidelberg in 1977, and later was hired to edit a book on women's reproductive health, written by the FFWHCs. The project eventually yielded two books: *A New View of a Woman's Body: An Illustrated Guide* and *How to Stay Out of the Gynecologist's Office*, both published in 1981.

The early editions of *Our Bodies, Ourselves* opened a tsunami of hitherto unavailable information about basic physiology and self-care, and provided sophisticated critiques of medical studies that enabled women to make truly informed choices about the diagnosis and treatment of common conditions, from yeast infections to cancer. I benefited enormously from this information, and working as a lay health worker in the clinic in Los Angeles provided an even deeper level of knowledge and skills. Through my work on both the books and my work in the clinic, I gained new insights into abortion, birth control, vaginal health, sexuality, childbirth, donor insemination, hysterectomy, and the highly charged politics of women's health. As I talked to women about their health concerns, it was not only enormously gratifying to be able to provide information that was often desperately needed, but to offer these clinical services on a woman-to-woman basis. In the clinic, we provided in-depth information, and I noticed that clients were often relieved that we *weren't* gynecologists. We did most of our health care in groups, teaching breast self-exam, showing women our cervixes before we helped them see their own, and giving out plastic speculums as freely as other businesses distribute ballpoint pens. We taught our doctors how to perform abortions using the smallest possible instruments to minimize discomfort and allow the procedure to be done without anesthesia. We established a later abortion hospital program that served women from the western United States, Canada, and Mexico; taught ourselves to fit cervical caps; and started the first donor insemination program outside of a commercial sperm bank. We gave papers and workshops at conferences such as the National Women's Studies Association, the American Public Health Association, Planned Parenthood, and the National Abortion Federation. Staff members traveled to Mexico, Central America, Europe, and the Middle East to meet feminists who shared our concerns. And we published our books.

After leaving the FFWHCs, I moved to New York City and began writing books about women's health, including *The Complete Cervical Cap Guide,* and collaborating on books like *Overcoming Bladder Disorders* and *A Woman's Book of Choices: Abortion, Menstrual Extraction, RU-486.* I also lectured at universities and women's groups across the country and spoke at sexuality conferences around the globe, including the

First International Conference on Orgasm in New Delhi, and the World Congress of Sexology in Heidelberg, Yokohama, and Hong Kong.

After finishing *A Woman's Book of Choices*, I began working on a proposal for a book on women's sexuality. The book, as I envisioned it, would introduce the FFWHCs' stunning reinterpretation of women's genital anatomy to a wider audience, investigate how this information got lost, and explore why this information is so vital to our understanding of women's sexuality. As my work progressed, I found out how the tiny glans came to be considered the clitoris and why women's sexuality is defined by male standards, what I've come to call the "male-centered, heterosexual model of human sexuality." Finally, I really understood what my colleagues at the FFWHCs and other feminist sexuality activists had discovered early on: sex was not going to improve for women until they began exploring and defining their sexuality for themselves. We need more than contraception and a public discussion of sexuality that the limited sexual revolution of the 1960s provided. (I say "limited," because the sexual revolution of the 1960s liberated men's sexuality more than it did women's.) What we need is a new vision of sexuality that encompasses women's needs, abilities, problems, and preferences.

I also started to read professional sexuality literature and sex advice books. One day, in preparation for a lecture on the history of sexuality, I made a list of the ways in which feminists had already begun to revise the male-centered, heterosexual model. To my surprise, the list included well over a dozen specific areas in which major changes had already occurred. The feminist sexual revolution, I belatedly realized, had already started, and the theme of my book suddenly became clear!

The Clitoral Truth provides information about women's sexual response that has long been dismissed, undervalued, unexplored, or misunderstood. This in-depth exploration of women's genital anatomy and sexual response is intended to help women understand sexual sensations and discover how to enhance their sexual response, in a more concrete way than has any other sexuality advice book. Many women and their partners, both male and female, want to learn as much as they can about sexual response in order to discover new and more rewarding ways of experiencing and sharing pleasure. I know that the detailed depiction of our genital anatomy in *A New View* helped me to understand my own sexual response in a far more meaningful and useful way, and thousands of women and men who have attended lectures and workshops given by me and my former colleagues at the FFWHCs have agreed. The physiological information in this book is intended to render a more fully realized portrait of women's sexual response, one that will hopefully enable women to perceive the complexity, intensity, and rewards of their sexuality.

The Clitoral Truth also explores ways women are seeking to enhance their sexual response through masturbation, sex toys, videos, books, workshops, individual coaching sessions, and sexuality information available on the Internet.

The book is intended for a broad readership, from heterosexual women to lesbians, and anyone who has felt excluded from the male-centered, heterosexual model of sexuality. Without the groundbreaking work of feminists, many of whom worked unacknowledged for years, this model of sexuality would remain firmly in place, and this book could not have been written. One of the most exhilarating things my research has revealed is that many of the changes that have contributed to the genuine sexual revolution for women were driven by feminists, and I am proud to call myself one.

Most medical dictionaries and textbooks describe the penis in glorious and meticulous detail, usually with informative illustrations. The clitoris, portrayed as the glans and a few associated parts, typically merits a brief paragraph, and usually lacks illustrations. If an illustration of the clitoris is included, it is often suggested by a little bump or a squiggly line surrounded by unnamed parts and white space. Using such truncated definitions and sketches, it is impossible to explain how women experience sexual response and orgasm.

For more than 2,500 years the clitoris and the penis were considered equivalent in all respects except their arrangement. After the eighteenth century, however, this knowledge was gradually suppressed and forgotten and the definition of the clitoris shrunk from an extensive organ system to a teeny pea-sized bump. The full extent of the clitoris was alluded to by Masters and Johnson in 1966, but in such a muddled fashion that the significance of their description became obscured. That same year, feminist psychiatrist Mary Jane Sherfey published an article about female sexuality that fleshed out the clitoris, as it were, and in 1981, the FFWHCs completed this process with anatomic precision.

The first chapter of *The Clitoral Truth* defines the male-centered, heterosexual model of sexuality, and determines what women have lost by having their sexuality defined against it. The heart of this chapter—and indeed the heart of the book—is a walking tour through our largely unknown genital anatomy based on the FFWHCs' definition. During our tour, we will explore every nook and cranny of this fabulous organ and see how its many surprising parts work together to produce orgasms. From there, we will travel through history to learn how women's genital anatomy has been defined through the ages to discover how such critical information about women's anatomy got lost.

In recent years, the issue of female ejaculation has become a source of controversy among feminists, sexologists, and the general public. Initially the concept may seem wildly audacious, intended more to inspire debate than to impart knowledge, but, as we will see in chapter 3, there is a sound anatomical basis for female ejaculation. Here you will meet women who ejaculate, in personal accounts that illuminate in explicit detail both how they experience it and how they feel about it. We will also visit the lost history of female ejaculation, discovering that it has, in fact, been described in the earliest sexuality advice manuals, and discussed in medical literature since the time of the ancient Greeks.

In addition to providing a more concrete understanding of women's genital anatomy and sexual response, we will bear witness to the ways in which women have begun to transform male-centered sexuality by rewriting the intercourse "script" and expanding "sex" to include far more than penis-in-vagina sex play. In the 1970s, feminists salvaged masturbation from thousands of years of religious condemnation, promoting it as both a legitimate and primary act of self-loving, one of the key elements in women's sexual self-discovery, and a component of partner lovemaking. In the section "A Short History of Masturbation" in chapter 4 (see page 141) we will also explore the history of social taboo, as well as religious and official sanctions against self-pleasuring, and see how women today are using vibrators, dildos, and other sex toys and fantasies to heighten their sexual experiences.

Finally, we will see how we can expand the definition of sex from the standard foreplay-intercourse ideal to a far broader concept of sexuality that emphasizes full-body pleasure. You will meet women who have attended workshops designed to help actualize this goal, and I will share the positive experiences I've had.

The task of transforming the male-centered model of sexuality and developing a more equitable ideal is a challenging endeavor. It requires, in part, reclaiming information about women's bodies and sexual response that has been lost or ignored under the antique phallocentric model. It also demands a broader understanding of what sexuality is and isn't, that it isn't just mood, body parts, revealing underwear, and orgasms. It's a part of who we are as sentient human beings, and it varies from person to person, culture to culture. Constructing a new model requires a thorough evaluation of the psychological, social, and biological facets of sexuality.

While the larger part of sexuality is certainly psychological, *The Clitoral Truth* focuses on the physical aspects of pleasure. The text and illustrations are designed to give women and their partners information, tools, resources, and ideas about how to understand and expand their sexual interests and potential. To create a more equitable framework for the physical elements of sexuality, men must modify their socialized model of stimulation-erection-ejaculation, which works very well for them, but has been shown in study after study to be far less effective for women. The key is that men must be willing to learn some degree of ejaculatory control. Perhaps the biggest step in constructing a new vision of sexuality is for women to develop a stronger sense of themselves as independent sexual beings and assume a sense of sexual agency that has for so long been solely the birthright of men.

This is not a relationship book, although many relationships may be sexually enlivened and deepened through use of the information it provides. It is a book about our physical bodies and the significant part they play in the larger symphony of sexuality.

THE CLITORAL TRUTH
There's More to the Clitoris Than We Ever Imagined! 1

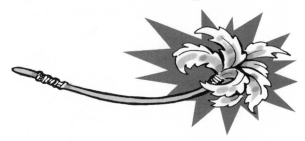

MALE-CENTERED SEXUALITY
A Full Frontal View

Despite three decades of activism since the 1960s, the perception of women's sexuality as less powerful, compelling, and profound than that of men is still almost universal. Since ancient Greece, men's bodies—with their sculpted muscles, visible genitals, and ready sexual response—have been perceived as the perfection of beauty. Set against this ideal, women's bodies—with their hidden genitals, softer flesh, and slower sexual response—have been viewed as imperfect. Today, men's sexual anatomy is still thought to be far more extensive and active than women's. Ejaculation and the single explosive orgasm are still seen as emblematic of men's superior sexual prowess, their sexual fantasies are thought to be more active and rewarding, and their need for sex more intense than women's.

From as far back as the Kinsey report in 1953, intercourse has not been found *not* to be the most effective means for women to experience the full range of their sexual response, and yet, penis-in-vagina sex remains ne plus ultra of sexual activity.[1] Other methods of achieving orgasm and sexual pleasure for women are considered second-rate, not "real" sex. If we learned anything from President Clinton and Monica Lewinsky, it's that most people still equate sex with intercourse. And men are seen as the sole possessors of the right to define and practice sex in ways that please them.

This male-centered concept of sexuality has been in existence for so long that we lack even the most basic vocabulary to describe our genital anatomy. Many women still think of their genitals as "down there" or make up pet names for them instead of directly referring to them with pride.

Most of today's sex advice books provide cartoon versions of women's genitals; *The New Joy of Sex* doesn't even have an entry for the clitoris. Even among anatomists and sexologists, there is an astonishing lack of agreement over what actually constitutes women's genital anatomy. Indeed, women's sexual expression has been profoundly suppressed by the male-centered intercourse ideal. Vaginal intercourse has been singled out as the only valid sexual activity, and heterosexuality has been promoted as the only genuinely approved norm. According to this line of reasoning, the sexual practices of lesbians and gay men are condemned as not "real" sex. Our concept of sex has become so male-defined that the single orgasm has become the gold standard for women's sexual response, and orgasm is often considered "optional" despite many women's ability to have multiple orgasms. In spite of countless historical references, studies, and anecdotal evidence, female ejaculation—the most dramatic of women's sexual secretions—is routinely dismissed by sexologists and physicians, and remains wildly controversial. It's no wonder that we often hear women's sexuality characterized as "mysterious," "perplexing," or "unknowable."

Clearly a revolution is in order. As I see it, this revolution must provide women with accurate and comprehensive information about their bodies and sexual response. Sexuality education and sex advice literature must offer a broader definition of what constitutes "sex," and promote a wider range of sexually pleasurable activities that enable women to have an equitable share of physically and emotionally rewarding sex. We must empower women to develop a stronger sense of self as social and sexual beings so that we may all be free to act assertively on our sexual desires. And finally, we must investigate the many social and psychological facets of sexuality to better understand their place and value in our lives.

A DEARTH OF WORDS

We've looked at sex through the phallocentric lens for so long that we don't even have a vocabulary to describe our genital anatomy and articulate sexual experiences. Psychologist Carol Tavris writes that "in spite of living in a culture that seems sexually obsessed, many women still do not even accurately name their genitals. At best, little girls are taught that they have a vagina, which becomes the word for everything 'down there'; they rarely learn they also have a vulva and clitoris. (Men have many words for their genitals, and none of them are vague.)" Tavris quotes writer Lucy Bland, who observes that "we face a past and a present in which there has never been a *language* allowing us to think about and define women's sexuality."[2]

A passage from *The Diary of Anne Frank* dated March 24, 1944—initially censored by Anne's father—poignantly illustrates the struggle that many women of all ages endure while trying to understand their bodies and their sexuality.

> I'd like to ask Peter [Peter Van Daan who, along with his family, joined the Franks in hiding in the Secret Annex] whether he knows what girls look like down there. I don't think boys are as complicated as girls. You can easily see what boys look like in photographs or pictures of male nudes, but with women it's different. In women, the genitals, or whatever they're called, are

hidden between their legs. Peter has probably never seen a girl up close. To tell you the truth, neither have I. Boys are a lot easier. How on earth would I go about describing a girl's parts? I can tell from what he said that he doesn't know exactly how it all fits together. He was talking about the "*Muttermund*" (cervix), but that's on the inside, where you can't see it. Everything's pretty well arranged in us women. Until I was eleven or twelve, I didn't realize there was a second set of labia on the inside, since you couldn't see them. What's even funnier is that I thought urine came out of the clitoris. I asked Mother one time what that little bump was, and she said she didn't know. She can really play dumb when she wants to!... But to get back to the subject. How on earth can you explain what it all looks like without any models? Shall I try anyway? Okay, here goes!... When you're standing up, all you see from the front is hair. Between your legs there are two soft, cushiony things, also covered with hair, which press together when you're standing, so you can't see what's inside. They separate when you sit down, and they're very red and quite fleshy on the inside. In the upper part, between the outer labia, there's a fold of skin that, on second thought, looks like a kind of blister. That's the clitoris. Then come the inner labia, which are also pressed together in a kind of crease. When they open up, you can see a fleshy little mound, no bigger than the top of my thumb. The upper part has a couple of small holes in it, which is where the urine comes out. The lower part looks as if it were just skin, and yet that's where the vagina is. You can barely find it, because the folds of skin hide the opening. The hole's so small I can hardly imagine how a man could get in there, much less how a baby could come out. It's hard enough trying to get your index finger inside. That's all there is, and yet it plays such an important role![3]

Anne Frank, who died at Bergen-Belsen, a Nazi prison camp, just before her sixteenth birthday, is renowned for her precocity about culture, politics, and human nature. In this long-expurgated passage from her diary, we discover a young woman in total isolation who has no peer models or parental support, struggling to comprehend her sexual self. One gets the feeling that Anne would have been eager to learn about the interior, secret parts of the clitoris if only she had been afforded the chance. This passage reveals that she did know a tremendous amount about her genitals, which given the time, circumstance, and her age, is truly remarkable. Today most girls her age couldn't name half of these parts accurately.

As you will see, we will find this missing information so that we can have a vocabulary to describe our genital anatomy, make sense of our sexual experiences, discover how to enhance them, and understand where orgasms come from.

IN THE MID-1950S, GROWING UP in a small town in the South, my friends and I suffered from adult amnesia about sexuality and a dearth of words similar to Anne Frank's. When I was in the seventh grade, we had a one-hour "sex education" session. During this highly charged but rather unrevealing time, we watched an animated cartoon that depicted a sperm literally floating from the outline of a male body into the abdomen of the outline of a female body. As did most adolescents in the 1950s, we educated ourselves in haphazard, sometimes serendipitous ways. In the eighth grade, two of us babysat for our chorus teacher and quickly discovered a "marriage manual" on her bookshelf. The next time she and her husband went to a movie, a mixed group of five or six of us showed up as soon as the taillights of their car disappeared over the hill. Over the next few months, we read the "marriage manual" aloud from cover to cover, when-ever two of us babysat. We found out how to engage in foreplay, how the sperm really gets into the vagina, and how a man and a woman achieved simultaneous orgasm (in theory). But the vocabulary remained somewhat opaque. I remember being particularly flummoxed by the term "labia." There were no pictures in the manual, and the dictionary was useless, since I had no idea what "genitals" were.

Naturally, we wanted to know more, so we hatched a bold plan. After school, five or six of us took the city bus to the Florida State Library. I had been a regular library-goer since the fifth grade, and knew my way around the stacks. Having no sense that we were about to perform a radical act, but well aware that we were doing something "forbidden," we looked up

"Sex" in the card catalog and went immediately to the sexuality section. Naturally, the selection was limited, but we did find the Kinsey report, with its many accounts of real people having sex. A whole new world opened up for us. For me, the grand revelation was that this covert activity that provoked giggles, snickers, and knowing glances among adults, was indeed a ubiquitous, normal, and somehow intensely rewarding human activity. It was years, however, before I learned that "labia" meant "lips," which were not on the face but between a woman's legs on the face of the genitals. In retrospect, I now wonder if our teacher purposely left that book in plain view in her home to supplement the cartoon version of sexuality education we were given. For that era, it would have been a very subversive move.

In 1997, a bill providing the first-ever government funding for sexuality education from kindergarten through the twelfth grade was passed by Congress, and signed into law by President Bill Clinton. This would be something to celebrate if the bill had not been designed with input from conservative think tanks such as Focus on the Family and the National Association of Christian Education, which espouse abstinence until marriage as the only healthy sexual strategy. The bill provides $250 million over five years for programs that use medical misinformation and unproven psychological theories to promote fear and shame:

➡ Contraception: Young people may get sick or even die if they use it"
➡ STDs: Virtually no information is provided on how to prevent them
➡ Abortion: Exceedingly rare problems such as infection, hemorrhage,

future miscarriages, premature births, infertility, and post-abortion depression are presented as "very likely" outcomes

➡ Gender orientation: Homosexuality is depicted as "unhealthy"

➡ Nontraditional family structures are depicted as being "deeply troubled"[4]

All of this simplistic, sex-negative information is designed to discourage teens from engaging in sex. The bill expressly denies grants to any state or community whose programs contain any information or skill-training that helps teens develop positive attitudes toward sex and healthy sexual decision making and behavior. Certainly abstaining from intercourse until one is better equipped to handle the emotional and physical consequences is a valuable sexual strategy, but advocating abstinence as the only viable strategy leaves teens (more than 50 percent of whom are sexually active) vulnerable to the very real consequences of sexual involvement.

These government-funded programs, including Teen Aid and Respect, Inc., may actually be worse than what passed for sexuality education in the 1950s. In order to get useful, sex-positive information, young people are being forced, as they were in the past, to look outside of "sexuality education" for answers and solutions to their questions and sexual dilemmas. The lucky ones will find help. The unlucky ones will not, and there is a high likelihood that as they mature, they will view their sexuality through the sex-negative lens of the conservative eye. Fortunately those who do seek outside information have a plethora of options, a representative sample of which is listed in Resources beginning on page 213.

THE ANATOMY OF SEX

One of the reasons sex is thought to be more dynamic and rewarding for men than for women is that the penis is seen as much larger and more complex, and consequently more powerful, than women's genitals. After all, the penis is readily visible, usually snaps to attention at the drop of the trousers, and shoots off like a water pistol during orgasm. However, there is more to our genitals than meets the eye… or better yet, the hand.

The idea that the clitoris is as big and powerful as the penis may seem preposterous, especially if you look in almost any medical dictionary, anatomy text, or sexuality advice book and see a tiny glans labeled as "THE CLITORIS." So many books concur with the depiction of the clitoris as a miniscule pea, that one would be forced to conclude that this is true, and that those who think otherwise have a full-blown case of penis envy. But quite the opposite is true.

WHICH IS THE BOY AND WHICH IS THE GIRL?

If you were to look at an illustration of a human embryo at two months, it is impossible to discern the sex of the developing organism. During the first eight weeks of gestation, all embryos appear to be female. Around the seventh week, if the embryo has two X (female) chromosomes, it will continue to develop as a female. If it has one X and one Y (male) chromosome, it will begin to produce testosterone, which stimulates the growth of rudimentary male sexual features. So much for the Eve-out-of-Adam myth. As you can see, it is Adam-out-of-Eve. Figure 1 shows the common origins of the major parts of the male and female genital anatomy.

FEMINISTS REDISCOVER THE CLITORIS

The modern, anatomically correct definition of the clitoris was developed by the FFWHCs. None of the women in the group had any formal medical training, but they learned about basic well-woman gynecology by working in their clinics and reading widely in the field. In 1975, they decided to write a book on women's reproductive health using the knowledge they had gained through the day-to-day operation of their clinics. In addition to issues such as abortion, contraception, and vaginal health, they decided to include a chapter on sexuality.

"Initially, we thought we would just review the popular and medical literature on sexuality, critique it, and write the chapter, but we were in for a big surprise," says Carol Downer, the FFWHCs founder and its longtime CEO. "Little of what we found in sex advice books or in medical texts seemed to correspond to our sexual experiences or to illuminate them in any useful way."[5] They had run headlong into the male-centered, heterosexual model of sexuality.

In a quest to understand sexual response from a woman's perspective, nine women from the Los Angeles and Orange County, California,

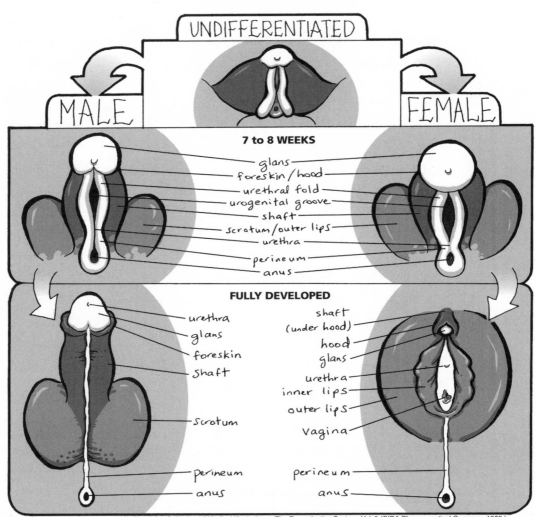

FIGURE 1: FETAL GENITAL ANATOMY

UNDIFFERENTIATED

MALE

FEMALE

7 to 8 WEEKS

- glans
- foreskin / hood
- urethral fold
- urogenital groove
- shaft
- scrotum/outer lips
- urethra
- perineum
- anus

FULLY DEVELOPED

- urethra
- glans
- foreskin
- shaft
- scrotum
- perineum
- anus

- shaft (under hood)
- hood
- glans
- urethra
- inner lips
- outer lips
- vagina
- perineum
- anus

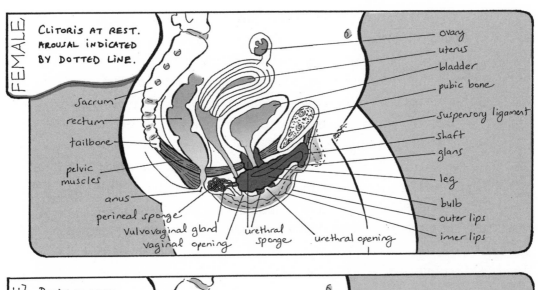

FEMALE

CLITORIS AT REST. AROUSAL INDICATED BY DOTTED LINE.

ovary
uterus
bladder
pubic bone
suspensory ligament
shaft
glans
leg
bulb
outer lips
inner lips

sacrum
rectum
tailbone
pelvic muscles
anus
perineal sponge
Vulvovaginal gland
vaginal opening
urethral sponge
urethral opening

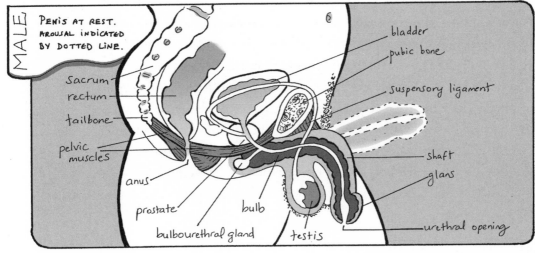

MALE

PENIS AT REST. AROUSAL INDICATED BY DOTTED LINE.

bladder
pubic bone
suspensory ligament
shaft
glans
urethral opening

sacrum
rectum
tailbone
pelvic muscles
anus
prostate
bulbourethral gland
bulb
testis

FIGURE 1a: FEMALE VS. MALE

FFWHCs—Carol Downer, Suzann Gage, Sherry Shiffer, Lorraine Rothman, Francie Hornstein, Lynn Heidelberg, Kathleen Hodge, Lynn Walker, and Chris Cleary—held regular consciousness raising sessions and shared their intimate sexual experiences in considerable depth. They dissected their sexual responses in minute detail, taking off their pants, sitting in a circle, and comparing parts of their visible genital anatomy to textbook illustrations. To find more detailed information, they examined classic anatomical illustrations, tracking down obscure references in eighteenth- and nineteenth-century European anatomy texts. The only modern book that they found to be illuminating was psychiatrist Mary Jane Sherfey's *The Nature and Evolution of Female Sexuality*.[6] Taking off from Masters and Johnson's definition of the penis, Sherfey argued that the clitoris is no more just its tip (the glans) than the penis is just its glans. She compared the clitoris to the penile anatomy point by point, demonstrating how they were equivalent to each another and finding the clitoris to be an extensive and powerful organ system.

Several women in the group made movies and took photographs of one another masturbating to closely observe the dynamic changes that occur in the visible structures of the clitoris during sexual response. In preparation for doing the anatomical illustrations, artist Suzann Gage, a member of the group, took an anatomy course at UCLA. Her illustrations vividly brought the group's concept of the clitoris to life.

Using historical and modern anatomical descriptions, the group enlarged and refined Sherfey's description of the clitoris, creating a new definition that encompassed all of the structures undergoing changes during orgasm, whether contributing to orgasm in a significant way or marking the boundaries. After doing their intensive study of women's genital anatomy, the FFWHCs identified eighteen structures; some of these are readily visible, while others cannot be seen but are easily felt, especially during sexual response. Still others cannot be felt, but when they are engorged with blood during sexual response, they cause the clitoris to greatly increase in size just as the penis does. The group's analyses and redefinition of the clitoris were originally published in a book I edited, entitled *A New View of A Woman's Body: An Illustrated Guide.*[7]

THE VISIBLE PARTS OF THE CLITORIS

The hairy outer lips (labia majora) are not considered a part of the clitoris because, embryologically speaking, they arise from the same fetal tissue as the scrotal sac, the pouch containing the testicles, which are a major component to the male reproductive system. The visible parts where the clitoris begins are found at the point—the junction or front commissure—where the edges of the outer lips meet at the base of the pubic mound. (The points where the corners of the eyelids and of the lips meet are also called commissures.)

The word "glans" comes from the ancient Greek word for "acorn," and was probably chosen because the tip of the uncircumcised penis with its foreskin pulled back looks somewhat like a ripe acorn peeking out of its cap. The clitoris has a glans as well: the exquisitely sensitive nub that is, without question, the crown jewel of the clitoral system. The female glans, however, has one surprising and exhilarating difference. It holds between 6,000 and 8,000 sensory nerve endings, more than any other structure in the human body—male or female—and by one estimate about four times as many as the glans of the penis. This hypersensitive little node has only one purpose: pleasure, and its ability to receive and transmit sensations of touch, pressure, and vibration is unsurpassed.

The glans may be the crown jewel of the clitoral system, but the hairless inner lips (or labia minora, Latin for "little lips") are typically the most prominent feature of the visible clitoris. The moist wings of tissue enfold the glans, the urethral opening, the vaginal opening, and the two ducts of the paraurethral glands on either side of the urethral opening. The appearance of the inner lips varies greatly from woman to woman. They may range in color from pale peach to mauve, burgundy, or dark chocolate and the color may deepen after childbirth. The lips may be very trim and narrow, curled inward, fluted, or so widely flared that they protrude past the pubic hair. Their texture may be smooth, glassy, almost translucent, or deeply crinkled. It is not uncommon for one lip to look quite dissimilar to its mate. Betty Dodson, who was an artist before she became a sex educator, likes to characterize the inner lips in artistic terms such as "classic," "gothic," "baroque," "art deco," and "modern." "They are like snowflakes," she says. "Every one is unique and beautiful."[8]

One of the important corrections that the FFWHCs made to the traditional definition of the clitoris was to change the names of the labia majora (big lips) and labia minora (little lips) to outer lips and inner lips. "In looking at our own genitals, and at hundreds of photographs that we took, we observed that 'big' and 'little' could be misleading," explains Carol Downer. "Quite often the 'little' lips (labia minora) might be very pronounced, while the 'large' lips (labia majora) might be relatively slim... This more accurately describes what you actually see." It's interesting that in her intuitive description of the external genitalia, Anne Frank (see pages 24–26) uses the terms "outer labia" and "inner labia" instead of "big" and "little."

The outer edge of each inner lip flares and continues toward the pubic mound (*mons veneris* in Latin, or Mound of Venus), forming a protective hood over the glans. The hood is analogous to the foreskin of the penis. The inner edges of the inner lips meet just underneath the glans, forming an upside-down "V." This point is called the bridle, or frenulum. The inner lips are richly endowed with nerve endings,

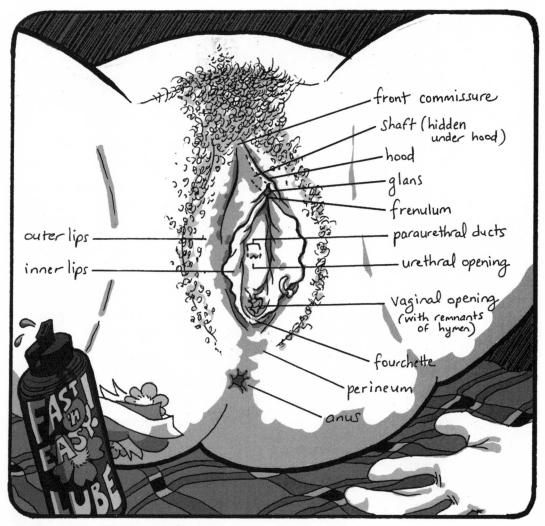

FIGURE 2: THE VISIBLE PARTS OF THE CLITORIS

making them quite sensitive to sexual stimulation. Some women say that their inner lips are actually more sensitive than the glans.

The bottom edges of the inner lips meet just beneath the vaginal opening, forming an opaque membrane—the little fork, or fourchette, which represents the lower boundary of the visible portion of the clitoris. The fork may be torn or cut during childbirth, and its appearance may change or it may be obliterated altogether. Like the commissure that marks the upper extent of the visible clitoris, the fork marks the lower boundary.

If you separate the inner lips and stretch the vaginal opening slightly, you may be able to see the remnants of the hymen. At birth the hymen is stretched across the vaginal opening, but it is often frayed, torn, perforated, or it simply disintegrates by the time a woman reaches her mid-teens. For much of history, the intact hymen has been emblematic of a woman's virginity, indicating that she has not been penetrated by a man's penis. This concept was established in early patriarchal cultures when women and children were considered property, and girls were sold into marriage in their early teens. A girl had to be a virgin and remain faithful during marriage in order for her husband to be assured that her children were also his children. Today, the essential fragility of the hymen would seem to make it an unreliable indicator of whether or not a woman has had intercourse. In rare cases, it is possible that a hymen may be elastic enough to admit a penis without tearing.

Figure 2 shows the visible parts of the clitoris as well as some non-clitoral structures: the outer lips, the urethral opening, where the urine comes out, the vaginal opening, and the perineum, the little bridge of skin between the vagina and the anus. If you have a mirror handy, you can easily locate these structures. While masturbating or having sex with a partner, you can observe how these parts change in size and/or color when you are excited.

The FFWHCs emphasizes the tremendous variation in the size and appearance of women's genitals. "Working in our clinics we observed a much wider range of 'normal' than was ever indicated in medical texts or even sex advice books," Downer said. "The implication was that if your genitals didn't look pretty much like those pictured, you were somehow abnormal. Our experience in the clinic suggested that this was wrong, and decided to set the record straight."[9] A group from the clinics, together with photographer Sylvia Morales, traveled around the country, taking more than a thousand photographs of women's genitals. "The enormous variation we observed in the appearance of the visible parts of the clitoris as well as the vulva, vagina, and cervix, convinced us that we were correct," Downer says. Eventually, a selection of these photographs appeared in *A New View of a Woman's Body*. Other photographs revealing the variety in the appearance in women's genitals can be found in *Femalia*, edited by Joani Blank. Drawings can also be found in Tee Corrine's classic *Cunt Coloring Book* and in Betty Dodson's *Sex for One* (see Resources).

In the proverbial locker room, men are known to compare their penises, and this behavior allows them a window into the range of what "normal" actually is. This isn't something that many women feel comfortable indulging in, and consequently they suffer intense isolation, wondering if they are "normal," or in some cases, if they even have a clitoris.

Now that we've explored the visible parts of the clitoris—you've studied the illustrations—you might want to take out a mirror and locate them for yourself. Keep in mind that these illustrations represent only a few of many possible variations in the size and appearance of the clitoris.

THE HIDDEN PARTS OF THE CLITORIS

If you were to remove the top layer of skin and visible structures of the clitoris, it would reveal numerous hidden structures, which Mary Jane Sherfey referred to as the "powerhouse of orgasm." These structures include erectile tissue, glands, muscles, blood vessels, and nerves. In both the clitoris and the penis, there are two types of erectile tissue: body of caverns *(corpus cavernosum)* and spongy body *(corpus spongiosum)*, which fill with blood during sexual response, causing an erection.

The clitoral shaft is attached to the glans, just underneath the surface of the skin. The shaft is a round fibrous segment of spongy erectile tissue, and like the glans, it is very sensitive. If you roll your finger back and forth just above the glans during sexual response, you should be able to feel a hard ridge about one-half to one inch long, and about the diameter of a soda straw, and rises toward the pubic mound for a short distance, then bends sharply and divides, forming two slender legs or *crura* (Latin for "legs"), which are also composed of spongy tissue. The legs of the clitoris flare out somewhat like the wishbone of a chicken.

If you look at Figures 3 and 4, you will notice that underneath the inner lips are twin bulbs of cavernous erectile tissue. During sexual response these structures fill with blood, which then becomes trapped in their cryptic spaces, causing erection.

In both women and men, the urethra (the tube through which we urinate), is surrounded by a ring of spongy erectile tissue that is identical to the type of erectile tissue, *corpus spongiosum*, that surrounds the penis. In women, the urethra is about two inches long, and runs from the bladder to the urethral opening just above the opening to the vagina. "In nearly all of the modern anatomy books that we looked at, the erectile tissue surrounding the urethra was missing," Carol Downer says. "Although it is clearly analogous to the spongy tissue which surrounds the urethra in men, it hasn't been considered a part of the clitoris for several hundred years. Since it had no name in women, we decided to name it the urethral sponge."

The urethral sponge is a very significant part of the clitoral system. Embedded in its spongy erectile tissue are up to thirty or more tiny prostatic-like glands that produce an alkaline fluid similar in its constitution to the male prostatic fluid. Two of the largest, called Skene's glands, are near the urethral opening, where the urine comes out, but numerous others are buried in the spongy tissue surrounding the urethra. All of these glands together are referred to as paraurethral glands, meaning "around the urethra," and they are the source of female ejaculation. Normally, the sponge is collapsed and is difficult to feel, but during sexual response, if you or your partner puts a finger in your vagina and presses toward the pubic mound, you can feel a rough nugget about the length of the first one or two finger joints; that is the urethral sponge. When the sponge is filled with blood, i.e., erect, many women find that it is extremely sensitive to stroking, thrusting, or vibration inside of the vagina. The "G spot" is located on the part of the urethral sponge that can be felt through the vaginal wall. We'll look at this intriguing part of the clitoris in detail in chapter 3.

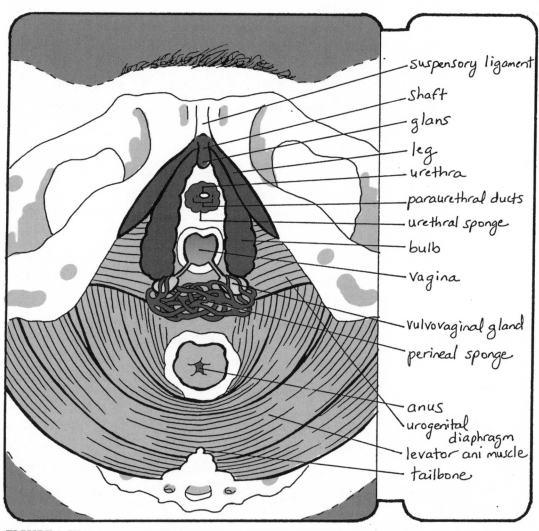

FIGURE 3: THE HIDDEN PARTS OF THE CLITORIS (FULL ON VIEW)

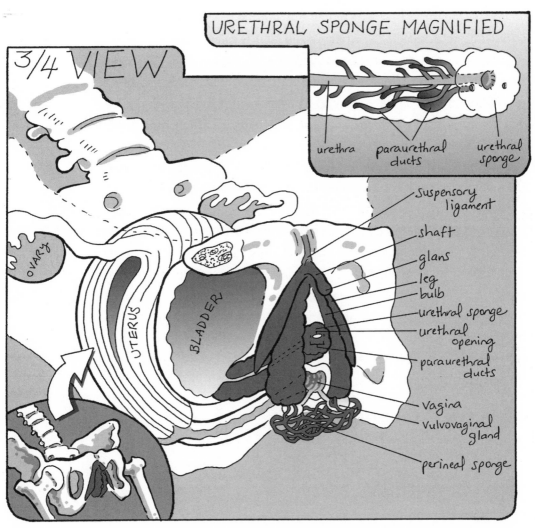

FIGURE 4: THE HIDDEN PARTS OF THE CLITORIS (3/4 VIEW)

Inside the inner lips, just below the vaginal opening, there are the all-but-invisible ducts for two bean-sized glands called the vulvovaginal, or Bartholin's glands. During sexual response, these small glands produce a few drops of rather thick viscous fluid, which contributes to lubrication of the vaginal opening. The amount of fluid produced can vary from woman to woman, but it is usually so small that it goes unnoticed.

Underneath the perineum, the short bridge of tissue between the fork, which marks the bottom boundary of the clitoris and the anus, is a dense network of blood vessels, often labeled in anatomy texts—if it is labeled at all—as the "perineal body." During sexual response, this tightly packed tangle of blood vessels fills with blood like the other erectile tissues do, becoming hypersensitive to touch, pressure, and vibration. Many women and men find that the perineum is intensely sensitive during sexual response and that stimulation or pressure on this area can often be felt deep inside the abdomen. Since this structure was rarely shown or labeled in anatomy texts, the FFWHCs named it the perineal sponge.

THE PELVIC FLOOR MUSCLES

The clitoris has several layers of muscles often referred to as the "vaginal muscles," but they are more correctly referred to as the "pelvic floor muscles." (See Figure 5.)

The oval-shaped bulbocavernosus muscle lies between the inner lips and the bulbs of the clitoris, which are composed of cavernosus erectile tissue, and it mimics their shape; hence its name. Both the vagina and urethra pass through this muscle. At its bottom, the bulbocavernosus muscle is interwoven with the anal sphincter muscle, which encircles the anus. Together, these muscles form a figure eight. Knowing that muscles surrounding the clitoris and the anus are connected to one another helps us to understand why anal stimulation feels good, and that it is an integral part of sexual response.

Underneath the glans, the ischiocavernosus muscles flare out on either side, sandwiched between the legs of the clitoris and the bulbs, like an upside-down "V." The bottom ends are attached to the ischium bones (the bones that we sit on). The transverse perineal muscle stretches like a fat rubber band from side to side, attached to the ischium bones on both ends and interwoven with the bulbocavernosus and anal sphincter muscles at the center. This wide band of muscle is so named because it transverses beneath the perineum, the short bridge of skin that separates the vagina and the anus.

The urogenital diaphragm is a flat, triangle-shaped muscle that is outlined by, and lies underneath, the ischiocavernosus and transverse perineal muscles. Both the urethra and vagina pass through this muscle.

Underneath everything lies the broad, flat, funnel-shaped sheet of muscle, the levator ani. The levator ani, better known as the pubococcygeus or "PC" muscle, is a part of the pelvic diaphragm. The urethra, vagina, and anus all pass through this muscle, which forms the absolute bottom of the pelvic floor.

There are two ligaments that play a role in sexual response. One end of the suspensory ligament is attached to the glans; at the other end it branches and attaches to the ovaries. During sex this ligament, which is like a big rubber band, tightens, pulling the glans back underneath its hood. This is why the glans is often harder to see or feel as you become more sexually excited. The ends of the round ligament are woven into the soft tissue underneath the inner lips, and the other ends are firmly attached to the uterus. This is why the uterus is affected by and is involved in sexual response.

Sensory messages are carried from the clitoris up the spinal cord to the brain and back by the pudendal nerve. Pudendum means "shame" in Latin. I would appeal to anatomists to come up with a more positive and descriptive name for this major nerve—something like, for example, the genital nerve, or the primary genital nerve, if research confirms that there is more than one major nerve complex serving the genitals.

Last, but far from least, are the blood vessels. In response to normal stimulation, arteries bring an increased blood supply to the clitoris, engorging the erectile tissues, causing erection, and setting the stage for orgasm. Veins then carry blood out of the clitoris. A study by Ital-

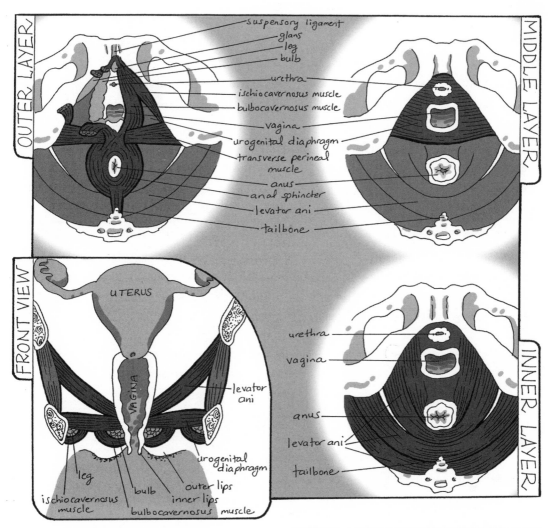

suspensory ligament
glans
leg
bulb
urethra
ischiocavernosus muscle
bulbocavernosus muscle
vagina
urogenital diaphragm
transverse perineal muscle
anus
anal sphincter
levator ani
tailbone

FRONT VIEW

UTERUS

VAGINA

levator ani

urogenital diaphragm

leg
ischiocavernosus muscle
bulb
bulbocavernosus muscle
outer lips
inner lips

urethra
vagina
anus
levator ani
tailbone

FIGURE 5: THE PELVIC FLOOR MUSCLES

ian anatomists has suggested that erection may be somewhat different in men than in women. In men, the blood rushes into the penis, trapped by the contraction of the pelvic muscles until it is released through a dense network of veins called a venous plexus and by the spasms of orgasm. Blood also rushes into the clitoris, and it too greatly increases in size, but, these researchers found, there is no concentrated venous plexus, so the blood flows out more readily. According to these researchers, this explains women's ability to experience multiple orgasm. It doesn't take such an explosive force to flush the blood out of the erectile tissues, and it refills again quickly, allowing for that second, tenth, or *nth* orgasm. Certainly erection does occur in women, but perhaps not as dramatically as it does in men. During full-blown sexual response, clitoral tissues expand enormously. The erectile tissues fill with blood, causing the clitoris to protrude enough, as one woman put it, "to fill my cupped hand."

DURING childbirth the perineum, perineal sponge, clitoral muscles, and vaginal floor are routinely cut— a procedure known as an episiotomy—to facilitate the passage of the baby through the vagina, and to avoid tearing. This cut to enlarge the birth canal goes through clitoral structures, most often the pubococcygeus (PC) muscle and the perineal sponge,

but sometimes through others as well. Some women find a decrease in sexual sensation after an episiotomy. Certainly more episiotomies are required today because of the use of painkillers and other practices designed to speed up birth, but we know from countries such as Holland and Germany where most births are still done by midwives that most episiotomies are unnecessary if childbirth is allowed to take its natural course and the perineum is properly prepared to stretch by warming and massage. Since clitoral tissues are cut, some midwives and childbirth educators believe that the episiotomy might be more properly be termed "clitorotomy." Perhaps obstetricians would cut less often and be more careful where they cut if they were aware that they are cutting through genital tissues, and that this may have a negative impact on a woman's sexual function afterward.

THE COMPLETE CLITORIS

All of the parts of the clitoris function together to provide sexual pleasure and orgasm, but the clitoris is certainly more than the sum of its parts. Women can experience sexual pleasure and/or orgasm without knowing anything about their anatomy, or indeed, without touching any part of it. But knowing that there is so much more to the clitoris than just the glans should lead us to the path of discovery about our potent sexual potential.

WHAT HAPPENS DURING SEXUAL RESPONSE AND ORGASM

Once, at a workshop on the clitoris that I had organized, Carol Downer was describing the various parts of the clitoris and how they all function to cause orgasms. As the slide showing the whole clitoris came on the huge screen, one woman in the audience let out an audible "ahhhhhhhhh!" After a few moments of dead silence, the entire room, crammed with more than three hundred people, erupted into applause and sympathetic laughter. When the laughter subsided, I realized that the proverbial lightbulb had flashed on in her brain, and she finally understood what must have previously mystified her, and so many women through the ages: where all of those exquisitely pleasurable sensations come from and how orgasm occurs.

As a prelude to sexual response, the senses make a subtle but profound and ultimately transformative shift from normal everyday cognitive function into the rarefied sphere of sexuality. Whereas moments before, the mind may have been occupied with the requirements, pleasures, or minutiae of daily life, the pleasure agenda suddenly demands to be fulfilled. Fantasies may invade the consciousness. We may touch our partner in ways and places that a scant minute ago would have been considered inappropriate, or we may reach for a vibrator. In response to this change in consciousness, the brain floods the bloodstream with more than a dozen feel-good hormones and sexual chemicals. While this phenomenon is largely unconscious, how we choose to act from this point forward determines what happens next. If, for example, we are in class or on the job, we might enjoy the promise of pleasure and surreptitiously masturbate, or save it for another time. If the time is right, however, the sequence of pleasure unfolds. Blood rushes to the pelvis and fills the erectile tissues. Nerve cells in the genitals become excited. The breasts may also increase noticeably in size and stimulation of the nipples causes the production of the potent hormone oxytocin, which causes urgent tingling sensations in the genitals.

The skin on various parts of the body becomes hypersensitive. The glans pokes its enlarged head from beneath the hood. The shaft now feels like a big round rubber band. The legs stiffen and elongate. The eggplant-shaped bulbs puff up like thirsty sponges, tightly cuffing the vaginal opening and causing the vulva to expand outward. The rough ridges of the urethral sponge can now be felt easily through the roof of the vagina, and if nothing is in the way, its tip may become easily visible through the vaginal opening. Pressure from dilated clitoral blood vessels (congestion in the veins, or vasocongestion) surrounding

ACCORDING TO THE FFWHCS, THE COMPLETE CLITORIS CONSISTS OF EIGHTEEN PARTS:

1. the clitoral junction (or front commissure, the point where the outer lips meet at the base of the pubic mound, marking the upper extent of the visible clitoris).

2. the glans.

3. the inner lips, or "labia minora."

4. the hood.

5. the bridle, or frenulum, the point where the outer edges of the inner lips meet just below the glans.

6. the fork, or "fourchette," the membrane stretched above the point where the lower edges of the inner lips meet below the vaginal opening, marking the lower extent of the visible clitoris.

7. the hymen, or its remnants, which are visible just inside the vaginal opening.

8. the shaft, which connects the glans and the legs.

9. the legs, or crura, two elongated bodies of erectile tissue shaped like a wishbone.

10. the bulbs, two large bodies of corpus cavernosum erectile tissue corresponding to the single bulb of the penis.

11. the urethral sponge, a body of corpus spongiosum erectile tissue surrounding the urethra.

12. the paraurethral glands: the female prostate glands.

13. the vulvovaginal, or Bartholin's, glands, which produce a small amount of lubrication outside of the vagina.

14. the perineal sponge, or perineal body, a dense network of blood vessels that lies underneath the perineum.

15. the pelvic floor muscles:

a. the bulbocavernosus (BC) muscle, which lies underneath the bulbs of the clitoris and the anal sphincter (AS) muscle.

b. the ischiocavernosus (IC) muscles, which outline the triangular pelvic opening, or outlet, and are attached to the bones we sit on.

c. the transverse perineal (TP) muscle, the broad band of muscle that outlines the bottom of the pelvic opening and is interwoven with the intersection of the bulbocavernosus muscle and the anal sphincter muscle.

d. the urogenital diaphragm (UD), the flat, triangle-shaped muscle that lies under the pelvic opening.

e. the levator ani (LA) muscle, a part of the pelvic diaphragm, the broad, flat, funnel-shaped muscle that is the bottom of the pelvic floor.

16. the suspensory ligament and the round ligament.

17. the nerves: the pudendal nerve, or, as I prefer to call it, the genital nerve complex, and possibly the hypogastric nerve, which carries messages back and forth from the uterus.

18. the blood vessels, which bring a greatly increased blood supply to the pelvis during sexual response.

NOW THAT'S SOME POWERHOUSE!

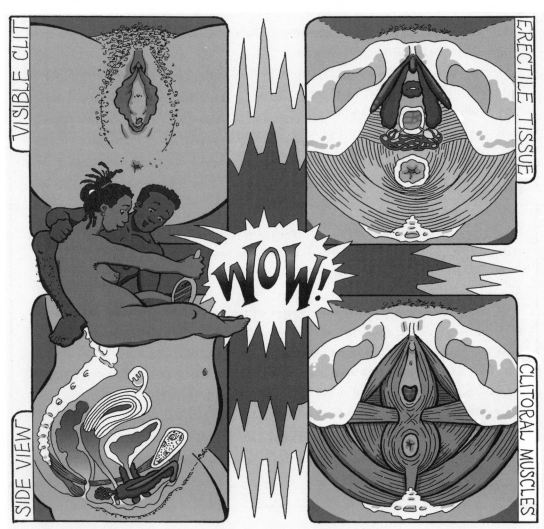

FIGURE 6: THE COMPLETE CLITORIS

the vagina forces clear fluid from the blood through the walls of the arteries and then through the walls of the vagina, producing the "vaginal sweat" that serves as a lubricant. This is not actually sweat containing urea and other waste products but a part of the blood serum. The vulvovaginal glands located near the base of the vaginal opening produce a small amount of a thicker viscous fluid, which also serves as a lubricant.

As stimulation continues, the muscles and ligaments begin to contract in response to messages from the brain, creating what we call "sexual tension." The suspensory ligament shortens and pulls the glans back underneath the hood, where it will probably remain until orgasm. (The glans can still be felt, but not as easily.) The end of the round ligament tugs on the inner lips on one end, and the uterus on the other, creating tension and pleasurable sensations in the inner lips and involving the uterus in the orgasmic process. In the meantime, muscle tension builds to a crescendo and all of the clitoral tissues become hypersensitive due to the increased blood supply. The bloodstream is now saturated with sexual chemicals and the skin on the rest of the body—the face and neck, abdomen, buttocks, hands, and feet—also becomes more sensitive, but you may hardly be aware of it, since the brain is now awash in naturally produced mind-altering substances. At some point, like an overloaded electrical circuit shorting out, the muscular tension explodes in a series of quick, rhythmic contractions, partially expelling blood from engorged tissues and releasing a further cascade of hormones, peptides, and opioids in the bloodstream and, ahhhhhhhhhhhh… orgasm!

Your orgasms may not seem like the idealized one described here. There are many different types: mini-orgasms; maxi-orgasms; quickie orgasms; explosive orgasms; multiple orgasms; dry, non-ejaculatory orgasms; extended orgasms, which can last anywhere from a few minutes to several hours; focused orgasms (experienced primarily in the genitals); irradiating orgasms, which may be felt in the pelvis and upper thighs; full-body orgasms; out-of-body orgasms (feels like it, anyway); well-earned orgasms; unconscious orgasms (the fabled "wet dreams," which may or may not involve genital engorgement and occur in both women and men); even involuntary orgasms, and so on. Sexologists generally agree that only the person experiencing an orgasm can adequately describe it. Therefore, the reasoning goes, only you can be the judge of the quality of an orgasm. In my view, there are no "bad" orgasms, just shorter, longer, weaker, stronger, and when time and circumstances permit, the much vaunted Vesuvian ones.

Beverly Whipple and Barry Komisaruk have proposed the concept of an "orgasmic process" in which sexual tension builds to a peak and orgasm occurs, followed by relaxation.[10] Having an orgasm, they say, is something like walking up a flight of stairs. Sequential steps must be taken in order to reach the top of the staircase. During sexual response, as sensory messages are sent toward the brain, increasing numbers of nerves become activated, reaching and then surpassing a threshold for activating another system. In other words, when one system reaches a certain peak of excitation, the nerve activity that it generates "recruits" or affects the next system along the chain. When all of the steps have been taken, and all of the systems are at a high level of excitability, they may reach a point of overload and discharge, causing an orgasm. These researchers also suggest that orgasms are most efficiently achieved if stimulation occurs "in phase" in a rhythmic cycle—what they call an "excitability cycle"—which is linked to the heartbeat: "The recruitment process possesses as an inherent property a rhythmically fluctuating level of excitability, i.e., an 'excitability cycle.'" This can be achieved, for men and some women, by the rhythmic thrusting of intercourse. For many women, as well as men, rapid hand movements, a vibrator, rhythmic leg motion, or other types of stimulation can create an effective excitability cycle that can result in orgasm. We know, of course, that orgasm can also occur without any of these types of mechanical stimulation.

This concept reveals, I think, why many women don't have orgasms all of the time. They simply aren't getting enough of the kind of stimulation and rhythm for a long enough time to recruit all—or enough—of the systems to cause an overload and explosive discharge of orgasmic energy. This is why masturbation is such an important learning mechanism. When we are by ourselves, perhaps aided by our favorite vibrator, some erotica, maybe some music, and anything else that helps us feel sexy and sexual, we can practice different types of stimulation for varying periods of time. If hands don't do the job, maybe a vibrator or other sex toy will. Given what I've learned about sexual response, I believe that any woman, from those who have never had an orgasm to those who are easily orgasmic, can have more and better orgasms by learning some basic anatomy and discovering what feels good.

Whipple and Komisaruk point out that their definition encompasses orgasms that are "characteristic of, but not restricted to the genital system." This is an extremely important feature of this definition, since feminists and sexologists have long promoted the concept of full-body sexual response and full-body orgasm, as opposed to the genitally focused orgasm, which has been the gold standard of male-centered sexuality.

A clear understanding of clitoral anatomy provides important information for women who have had their genitals mutilated (female genital mutilation, or FGM). In the less extreme version of female genital mutilation, only the glans is removed. In more drastic procedures, the glans, hood, shaft, and inner lips may be

excised and the edges of the outer lips sewn together with small openings left to drain urine and menstrual blood. The job is often done with dull, unsterile instruments. In the best-case scenario, where just the glans is excised, women may suffer decreased sexual sensation but they are still able to have orgasms. In the more radical forms of mutilation, however, women may develop infections that can be chronic or life-threatening, painful, or may restrict movement. Some women may also experience searing pain during intercourse. During each childbirth, the incision must be cut to allow for passage of the baby, and then resewn. Birth-related risks to both mother and infant increase dramatically. Cultures that place a high premium on virginity rationalize this ancient ritualistic practice as essential to discourage young girls from losing their virginity and becoming unmarriageable. Though the practice is intended to preserve a girl's virginity, it actually decreases fertility and reproductive ability. Genital mutilation does not prevent her from wanting to have sex, either. We now know that the biggest part of sex is psychological and hormonal. Thus, it is impossible to control the desire for sex through surgery, unless you remove part of the brain. And knowing what we now know about the extent of the clitoris, it is clear that no matter how is removed, the erectile tissues, glands, muscles, and nerves that are involved in sexual response cannot be diminished. Even women who have had the most severe mutilation still have "the powerhouse of orgasm" intact, and if their pain is not too great, they should still be capable of experiencing a wide range of sexual response—even orgasms. The same may be true for people who have had their genitals altered through illness or accidents.

A precise understanding of the extent and function of the genitals might also be enormously helpful to women and men who are exploring transgender roles or identities, or who are considering gender reassignment surgery. Until recently, surgery was thought to be essential for many transsexuals. Today, it is understood that the genitals are only one factor—and not even the most significant factor—in gender identity. As a consequence, a wider, more fluid continuum of gender identities has evolved that enables many people to find comfortable sexual personas without surgery. Knowing that women, men, and even those who have ambiguous genitalia have essentially the same genital structures arranged in one way or another, could be useful information for people contemplating gender reassignment surgery.

Over the years, I've explained the clitoris in self-help groups, classrooms, and at conferences and public forums. The reception has been overwhelmingly positive. These presentations always generate lively discussions, set off the proverbial lightbulbs, and in many cases transform the way that women think about sexual response and, ultimately, their sexuality. I asked a few women who have attended these sessions to describe the impact that this information has had on their thinking.

Tamara found an alternative to vigorous stroking: "After seeing the picture of a woman feeling the clitoral shaft, I experimented with rolling my finger slowly back and forth over it as I get lost in a fantasy. Now 'rolling the shaft' is one of my favorite sensations during sex." Kimeka discovered a new area where stimulation was uniquely effective: "Those visual images from *A New View of A Woman's Body* helped me focus stimulation in areas, such as the perineum, that I hadn't paid much attention to before. When my girlfriend applies slow, rhythmic pressure with her fingers or knuckles, I can feel it all the way up to my uterus. It really enlarged the area in which I feel sensations."

Cynthia found that something she thought was a problem wasn't really a problem after all: "I was already pretty self-aware, but seeing pictures of the whole clitoris made it crystal clear to me how my sexual arousal developed and why I was feeling things in certain places. Also it cleared up one really perplexing question. I had always had trouble urinating after orgasm, and I would try to force the urine out, but learning that the urethra is surrounded by erectile tissue helped me to see why you wouldn't be able to urinate right away and why that's all right."

Unlike Anne Frank's mother—and millions of other girls' mothers —Cynthia is able to give clear, useful answers to her daughter's questions about what's "down there": "Knowing the names and functions of all of the clitoral parts has allowed me to feel so comfortable helping my five-year-old learn about her genitals. I can give concrete answers with assurance and I feel very joyous about being able to pass this information on."

Andrea, who had never had an orgasm until she was in her mid-thirties, started masturbating and finally discovered what wasn't happening, became orgasmic, and then multi-orgasmic:

No matter how attracted I was to men, I never had an orgasm. I got lots out of affection, skin contact, fun, sometimes achieving a choice "conquest," but never orgasms. When I started having sex with women, I found out how much you could do to your partner with your hands, and sex reached a new level for me, but still... no orgasms. Then I started experimenting on myself. I found *A New View of a Woman's Body* and seeing how all those parts worked together gave me the necessary clues. Here's how I had my first orgasm: I planned what I was going to do all day and sort of talked myself into being excited. After dinner, I took a nice hot bath, put on my favorite opera CD, lit some candles, and got into bed. As I was masturbating (I had not graduated to vibrators yet), I thought about every single part of my clitoris. I slowly massaged the parts I could touch one at a time, thinking how it was changing and how it was connected to the next one. I could feel when things became engorged. My vulva puffed out, my lips were all tingly, my glans was very hard, and I could feel the shaft quite easily. Feeling with my hands what was going on was new to me. I experimented with different kinds of strokes on different parts; then quite by accident I found the one that worked. I put my index and middle fingers into my vagina curving them around under the pubic bone and used hard, fast strokes pulling the glans down and the inner lips in. I visualized the clitoral muscles and could feel them getting tighter. Then I had my first orgasm! I didn't feel spasms, but I felt this sort of golden glow in the clitoris that spread through my pelvis and down my legs like warm honey. My legs felt weightless and for maybe twenty seconds—who can tell time in this situation—my feet sort of went spastic.

Then, without warning, I burst into tears. I guess they were tears of relief. I kept masturbating and after a while I was able to have an orgasm with a partner. After a couple of years, I got more confident and started having up to a dozen orgasms during masturbation, but during sex with partners, I have to have help or give them to myself.

These are only a few of the personal experiences that women have related to me. They reveal the usefulness of clitoral literacy and suggest ways this information can be put to use in your own life.

WHY THE VULVA ISN'T THE CLITORIS

When most people think of women's genitals, they typically think of the vulva, the outer and inner lips, and the clitoral glans. In Latin, vulva means "wrapping" or "covering," and these definitions are certainly better terms than pudendum. The Romans used pudendum to refer to both the male and female genitals, and it is still used today in medicine to refer to the visible genitals of women. Traditionally, the vulva includes the hairy pubic mound and outer lips as well as the inner lips, and the introitus, or vestibule, the space around the vaginal and urethral openings. Some definitions of "vulva" include most of the visible structures. One I found also includes the clitoral bulbs. "We chose to exclude the outer lips from our definition because they are not particularly sensitive compared to clitoral structures which are richly endowed with nerve endings, and they do not undergo much change during sexual response," Carol Downer explains. "We also excluded the vestibule, the area around the vaginal opening encompassed by the inner lips, because it's really a space created by anatomical arrangement—it's not an anatomical structure." She also notes that the outer lips do not arise from clitoral tissue in the embryo, but from the "labio-scrotal swelling," which also produces the scrotal sac, which is an important reproductive structure in the male.

There is no male equivalent of the vulva. Classifying most of the clitoris as the vulva is like taking the male pubic mound and scrotum, adding the penile foreskin and glans, and calling it a "mulva," or "pulva," or something like that. It leaves out many crucial parts. Anatomists—and men—don't quibble about which parts belong to the penis. They *know*. The penis has an inviolable anatomic integrity that has not been accorded the clitoris—at least not since the Renaissance. Why do we tolerate such anatomic equivocation of women's genitals? In addition, defining the clitoris as "wrapping," "covering," or "vulva" implies passivity to women's genitals. This is not to say that the vulva is nonsexual. It's what a woman and her sexual partner see when they look at her genitals, what she first feels when she masturbates. Vulval structures—the pubic mound with its coarse pubic hair, and hairy outer lips—do have sensory receptors, but not in the dense

WOMEN CONCEPTUALIZE AND CHARACTERIZE THEIR ORGASMS VERY DIFFERENTLY. As well as anybody, and better than most, British poet Alison Fell captures the poignant diversity of the perception of women who shared their orgasmic experiences in consciousness-raising groups in the 1970s:

An orgasm is like an anchovy,
she says,
little, long, and very salty.

No, it's a caterpillar,
undulating, fat and sweet.

A sunburst, says a third,
an exploding watermelon:
I had one at Christmas.

Your body betrays, she says,
one way or another.
Rash and wriggling, it comes
and comes, while your mind
says lie low, or go.

Or else it snarls and shrinks
to the corner of its cage
while your mind, consenting
whips in and out, out in the open
and so free.

As for me,
says the last,
if I have them brazen
with birthday candles,
with water faucets
or the handles of Toby jugs,
I don't care who knows it.
But how few I have—
keep that in the dark. [11]

quantity that clitoral structures have. As one woman told me, "When I'm turned on, even my pubic hair is sensitive. I like my partner to run his hand or beard over it for a while before he touches anything else." Betty Dodson's video *Viva la Vulva* documents a group of women ages twenty-five to fifty-five sharing their feelings, exploring, and learning new things about both the vulva and the clitoris. This video, listed in Resources, is an essential primer for any woman who wants to become more intimately acquainted with the visible parts of her sexual anatomy.

WHAT HAPPENED TO THE VAGINA?

If you accept the definition of the clitoris described in this chapter, then you know that the vagina is not a part of it. Instead, the vagina is a major component of a woman's reproductive system. It provides an outlet for menstrual blood. The vagina also serves as a well-constructed receptacle for sperm, assuring perpetuation of the species. In addition, as the final portion of the birth canal, the vagina expands to at least ten times its normal size to allow for the passage of a baby.

In addition to its reproductive roles, the vagina does have specific sexual functions, but they are essentially passive. During the initial phases of sexual excitement, due to the pressure of increased blood volume, a colorless fluid filtered from the blood is pressed through the vagina's mucous membrane walls, creating the sensation of wetness, and providing lubrication that facilitates the insertion of the penis, fingers, vibrator, or other objects into the vaginal canal. This fluid, which is produced within one to two minutes of sexual stimulation, is known as "vaginal sweat"—the sexual secretion that is most familiar to us. The vagina provides access for direct stimulation of the urethral sponge, which runs along the top of the vagina. Many women do find vaginal penetration exquisitely pleasurable, and erroneously ascribe these sensations to the vagina. In reality, the sensations stimulated by penetration, whether with the penis, fingers, sex toys, or what have you, are caused by pressure on the parts of the clitoris that surround the vaginal opening—the clitoral bulbs; the wishbone-shaped legs, which encompass the bulbs like parentheses; the muscles through which the vagina and urethra pass; and the urethral sponge. When engorged with blood, these clitoral structures form a fat horseshoe-shaped cuff around the vaginal opening and are highly sensitive to touch, pressure, and vibration. The vagina does contain nerves that are responsive to pressure, so you may feel these sensations when something is pushed through the vaginal opening. The pressure of penetration may also cause pleasurable sensations in the perineal sponge, which is located just beneath the forward floor of the vagina. This "clitoral cuff" also provides the exact type of stimulation—friction and pressure—that men need to have an orgasm. As heretical as it sounds, in terms of sexuality, the vagina is more useful to men than it is to women!

SO WHAT TO CALL IT?

Many women have trouble saying "clitoris," as if it's a word in a foreign language. Well, in a way, it is. Its origin comes from the Greek word "*kleitoris*," meaning the female genitals. The preferred English pronunciation is KLIT-er-iss, but the secondary kli-TOR-iss is heard fairly often and is not incorrect. It's rather depressing to note that the clitoris is far better known by a host of derogatory euphemisms such as "pussy," "cunt," "twat," "snatch," or "beaver," among the hundreds of negative terms that have been commonly used over the years.[12] Even though the Greeks believed in the essential similarity of the male and female genitals, that does not mean that they had equal respect for them. The female genitals were the butt of jokes in countless plays, and "*cunnus*" or "cunt" appeared repeatedly in abusive graffiti. In recent years, feminists have sought to defuse the negative imagery conveyed by "pussy" and "cunt," recasting them with positive meaning, much as lesbians and gays have with the word "queer."

In contrast, the ancient Tantric and Taoist reverence for women's sexuality in general, and their genitals in particular, is illustrated by a host of lyrical euphemisms such as "Jade Gate" or "Jade Chamber," "Golden Furrow," "Anemone," "Pearl," "Oyster," "Lotus," "Lyre," and "Phoenix." The ancient Hindu term *yoni* has achieved some currency today, and has respectful, even worshipful connotations. Taken literally, *yoni* refers only to the vulva or the visible parts of the clitoris, and has never been used to encompass the greater, hidden parts of the female genitals. Because it is a foreign word, it serves as yet another euphemism for that word that is so hard for us to say. So what should we call "it"? I think it would be nice—to say nothing of anatomically correct—if we look at the female genitals and say in a strong clear voice: "clitoris."

Certainly there is far more to sex than erectile tissue, exotic hormones, and orgasms. There are also thorny, often intensely controversial social issues—and deeply complicated psychological ones—reproductive concerns, constantly shifting definitions of gender, and powerful, contradictory religious and spiritual constructs, all of which hinder our comfort with and enjoyment of sex. Yet, as I think this chapter reveals, the physical part of sexuality, especially of women's sexuality, has been profoundly misconstrued, misunderstood, and sadly neglected. At least we now know the *clitoral truth*: that women have a complex and powerful genital system that is designed for one specific purpose —*pleasure*. This knowledge should encourage us to explore our capacity for sexual response, and help us to do it with confidence and assurance.

THE CASE OF THE
MISSING CLITORIS
An Anatomical Detective Story

2

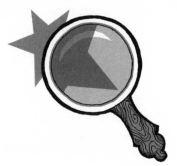

T he definition of the clitoris articulated by the FFWHCs always made perfect sense to me. But over the years, as I continued writing and lecturing about it, and telling women why looking at the clitoris as a complex and powerful organ is important, a question kept lurking around in the back of my brain. If the clitoris is equivalent to the penis in extent and power, how *did* this information get lost? I began to think that I was the only person on the planet who was curious about this question, but it seemed that it would take an enormous amount of research to track down the answer. As I read and scrounged for clues, the pieces of this puzzle began to fall into place, and a fascinating story emerged. This saga features some unlikely sleuths (a prominent history professor and two intrepid feminist sociologists), a host of respectable villains (some very famous European philosophers), a self-appointed world-class hit man (one Dr. Freud), and a bevy of accomplices (the vast majority of twentieth-century anatomists and sexologists). The drama details one of the grand heists of all time: the disappearance of women's genitals from anatomy texts, medical understanding, and popular perception. In a larger sense, it is the theft of women's right to comprehend, define, explore, and experience sexual pleasure on their own terms, rather than through male standards.

AN UNLIKELY DETECTIVE

In conducting a monumental study of the life cycle, Thomas Laqueur, Professor of History at the University of California at Berkeley, stumbled over the mysterious disappearance of women's genitals from anatomical illustrations quite by accident. In the introduction to his erudite and illuminating book, *Making Sex: The Body and Gender from the Greeks to Freud,* Laqueur describes his serendipitous encounter with a clue that led to his search for the answer:

I was on leave from St. Antony's College, Oxford, doing research for what was to be a history of the life cycle. I was reading seventeenth-century midwifery manuals—in search of materials on how birth was organized—but found instead advice to women on how to become pregnant in the first place. Midwives and doctors seemed to believe that female orgasm was among the conditions for successful generation, and they offered various suggestions on how it might be achieved. Orgasm was assumed to be a routine, more or less indispensable part of conception. This surprised me. Experience must have shown that pregnancy often takes place without it; moreover, as a nineteenth-century historian I was accustomed to doctors debating whether women have orgasms at all.... I discovered early on that the erasure of female pleasure from medical accounts of conception took place roughly at the time as the female body came to be understood no longer as a lesser version of the male's (a one-sex model) but as its incommensurable opposite (a two-sex model).[13]

Laqueur became intrigued and, as he describes it, his study of the life cycle "slowly slipped away." Harking back to the ancient Greeks, he set out to discover how, by the Victorian age, the clitoris had not only disappeared from medical texts and illustrations but how orgasm was banished from the Victorian concept of women's sexuality. Following is an outline of Laqueur's search for the lost clitoris and the culprits who did it in.

The Greeks believed that the male body was "perfect" and that the female body was an imperfect reflection of this ideal. In spite of this perceived lack of perfection, the Greeks clearly understood that the genitals of men and women were similar and functioned in a similar way to produce orgasm. Claudius Galen, the most famous physician of antiquity, was very straightforward about it: "All the parts, then, that men have, women have too, the difference between them lying in only one thing, namely, that in women the parts are within, whereas in men they are outside."[14] Galen argued that it was the greater heat of men that caused their genitals to protrude, and thus "perfected" them. In women, the cooler, imperfect sex, the genitals remained hidden from view. Laqueur calls this concept of equivalent genitals and equivalent sexual response the "one-sex" model.

Further, Laqueur's research reveals that the one-sex concept of equivalent genitals endured unchanged for more than 1,500 years, up to and throughout the Renaissance, and as a minority view during the eighteenth and nineteenth centuries.

RENAISSANCE MEN CONFIRM GENITAL EQUITY

The Greeks were so in awe of the human body that dissection was unthinkable. Most of what they understood about the genitals was inferred by their animal dissections. The Catholic Church, which dictated life in the Dark and Middle Ages, strictly forbade human

ALTHOUGH THE GENITALS WERE UNDERSTOOD to be equivalent, sex in ancient Greece was by no means equivalent for men and women. In the realm of the elite, men used sex to assert status and power over their inferiors: women, boys, slaves, and foreigners. Pleasure was a secondary goal. Women, who had no status to establish, were believed to be able to both give and receive pleasure. Men, in fact, believed that once women were aroused, they were insatiable, which presented a grave threat to the male-centered social order.

In an often quoted Greek myth, Hera, the queen of the Olympian goddesses, and her husband, Zeus, king of the Heavens, get into a furious row over who enjoys sex more, men or women. Hera asserts that it is men, while Zeus insists that it is women. In order to settle the disagreement, they decide to consult the sage Tiresias, who was known to have experienced sex as both a man and a woman. Tiresias agrees with Zeus, saying that women experience pleasure nine times more than men. Hera was so angry for losing the argument that she blinded poor Tiresias, who had only affirmed what Greek men believed about sex anyway.

dissection. Under the aegis of the church, medical research waned, but the masterworks of the Greeks remained available in surreptitious editions and served as the basis of rational medical knowledge until they were openly distributed again during the Renaissance.

Exploring and mapping the body was one of the grand obsessions during the Renaissance. In medical schools across Europe, the restrictions on human dissection loosened, opening the floodgates of discovery. The first anatomical illustrations of the human body were done in the late fifteenth century, and, as Laqueur notes, "the more Renaissance anatomists dissected, looked into, and visually represented the female body, the more powerfully and convincingly they saw it to be a version of the male's."[15] Echoing Galen in 1546, Charles Estienne, physician to King Louis XIV, confidently insisted that "what is inside women, likewise sticks out in males, but what is the foreskin in males is the pudendum [vulva] in women... what is a small covering [clitoral hood] in the opening of the vulva, such appears as a circular outgrowth [foreskin] of the male genitals."[16]

In the sixteenth century, the clitoris became the object of a famous Renaissance turf war between two preeminent Italian anatomists, Gabriel Fallopius and Renauldus Columbus. Each claimed to have "discovered" the clitoris. But Laqueur points out that "Kaspar Bartholin, the distinguished seventeenth-century anatomist from Copenhagen, argued in turn that both Fallopius and Columbus were being vainglorious in claiming the 'invention or first Observation of this Part,' since the clitoris had been known to everyone since the second century."[17] Fallopius succeeded, nonetheless, in having the egg transport tubes named in his honor, and today, we speak of the Fallopian tubes, although egg tubes would be a more descriptive and serviceable designation.

Laqueur explains that this knowledge of the entire clitoris was not the sole province of the intelligentsia. In a popular midwifery manual published in 1671, the English midwife Jane Sharp argued that the penis and the clitoris were nearly identical in structure and function. "The clitoris," she notes, "will stand and fall as the yard [penis] doth and makes women lustful and take delight in copulation."[18]

VIVA LA DIFFERENCE?

According to Laqueur, the one-sex concept remained intact until the eighteenth century when "sex as we know it was invented."[19]

Amidst the political ferment that led up to the French Revolution, women began to demand social and economic rights in salons, meetings, protests, and riots. Ironically, this was also the time when men began to "discover" significant sexual differences between themselves and women. "In the late eighteenth century, anatomists for the first time produced detailed illustrations of an explicitly female skeleton to document the fact that sexual difference was more than skin deep.

Where before there had been only one basic structure, now there were two," writes Laqueur.[20] The existence of specifically female nerve fibers was proposed. Most importantly, pregnancy and menstruation were now defined as illnesses that prevented women from playing a full and active role in society. Passion in women, who were weak from their maternal duties and functions, was classified as abnormal and considered properly replaceable by modesty. The role of sexual pleasure and orgasm for women began to be debated.

The leading philosophers of the day—the villains in our anatomical whodunit—abetted by men of the medical estate, concocted carefully crafted arguments for the sexual inferiority of women. The French philosopher Voltaire put it succinctly: "In physique, woman is weaker than man on account of her physiology. The periodic emission of blood that enfeeble women and the maladies that result from their suppression, the duration of pregnancy, the need to suckle infants and watch over them, and the delicacy of women's limbs render them ill suited to any type of labor or occupation that requires strength or endurance."[21] In Book Five of *Emile*, a social treatise disguised as a novel, Rousseau begins by "examining the similarities and differences between her sex and ours," arguing passionately that women were perpetually childlike and incapable of rational thinking.[22]

Although women were philosophically stripped of their right to passion and pleasure, the ancient fear of their sexuality remained. The

Greeks imprisoned their wives and condemned concubines and prostitutes to sexual slavery. Rousseau thought this a prudent idea, and believed, just as the Greeks did, that female reticence, discretion, and modesty really masked a fierce excess of passion that if unleashed, would disrupt the male-centered social order. Montesquieu pompously concurred, proclaiming in *The Spirit of Laws*, that "all nations agree in condemning female intemperateness."[23] And such statements from these prominent spokesmen were the veritable tip of the iceberg. Laqueur notes that "there were hundreds if not thousands of such works in which sexual differences were articulated in the centuries that followed." From this point on, women's sexuality was seen as very different from men's—increasingly weak, chaste, and passionless. Anatomists began to ascribe parts of the clitoris to the reproductive or urinary system. Medical illustrations became increasingly more simplistic, leaving parts of the clitoris unlabeled. By Victorian times, orgasm, which was previously accepted as a natural component of women's sexual repertoire, was seen as unnecessary, unseemly, perhaps even unhealthy for women. "The majority of women (happily for them) are not very much troubled by sexual feelings of any kind," the influential English urologist William Acton famously harrumphed.[24]

Although it was distinctly a minority view, not all anatomists agreed with the official concept of separate and unequal anatomies. In 1844 the German anatomist George Ludwig Kobelt published an exhaustive study of the clitoral system. His principle concern, Kobelt asserted, was "to show that the female possesses a structure that in all its separate parts is entirely analogous to the male." Citing the nineteenth-century view that women's genitals were insignificant, Kobelt insisted that "up to the present, the glans of the clitoris has been and still is considered a rudimentary, almost meaningless little structure." He later concluded that the function of the clitoris in sexual response "in accordance with its corresponding anatomical structure, can be no different than in the male." Alluding to the abysmal neglect of female sexual anatomy, Kobelt pointed out that at the time of his essay—mid-nineteenth century—the descriptions of certain parts of the clitoris had "completely disappeared from Physiology." Dismissing the eighteenth and nineteenth century views of women's sexuality as less passionate and rewarding than men's, Kobelt surmised that descriptions of women's genital anatomy would be remarkably different "if our physiological textbooks were in the hands of as many women," that is written by women, "as they are of men."[25]

DR. FREUD SHIFTS OFFICIAL FOCUS TO VAGINA

Sigmund Freud, the Viennese father of psychoanalysis, is the hit man who delivered the final blow to the concept of the multifaceted clitoris. Laqueur is certain that Freud was well aware of the anatomy of the clitoris as detailed by Kobelt and others. Yet, in his famous *Three*

Essays on Sexuality, Sigmund Freud insisted that the marvelous clitoris, which provides much unsupervised pleasure for young girls and adolescents, is "like a pile of pine shavings" useful only to "set a log of harder wood" i.e., the vagina, "on fire."[26] In other words, the clitoris is a child's plaything, while the vagina—the cozy space that has few nerve endings but provides such effective stimulation for the penis—is the grown-up woman's sexual destiny. This suggests that masturbation or other means of clitoral stimulation is an inappropriate or useless adult activity, and privileges heterosexual intercourse as the only healthy, mature, acceptable form of sexual activity for women. Freud's demotion of the clitoris and elevation of the vagina as the adult woman's primary means of giving and receiving sexual pleasure brought the male-centered heterosexual model of sexuality to its phallocentric apogee, and set in stone for the next century that it was not only appropriate but essential for women's sexuality to be defined in terms of male preferences.

Freud's summary dismissal of the clitoris as an important focus of sexual sensation for women had an atomic effect on how physicians and psychologists perceived women's sexuality. It was as if, for most of the twentieth century, women's extensive genital anatomy, and even the explosive little glans, was vaporized. Memory of the clitoris gradually faded until it became an anatomical nonentity.

In *Making Sex*, Laqueur makes the powerful and chilling argument that women's place in society is determined not by their anatomy and physiology, but by the way that their anatomy and physiology are defined and perceived. "Bodies, in these [Enlightenment] accounts are not the sign of but the foundation for civil society."[27] In other words, perceived differences in women's bodies became the rationale for denying them equal access to the social stage, just as perceived differences in their genital anatomy denied them the right to pleasure and orgasm in the eighteenth and nineteenth centuries. Thanks to Dr. Freud, this carried over through much of the twentieth century as well. Practically speaking, this means that as long as women's genitals are seen as inferior, our ability and right to explore and experience pleasure may continue to be seen as less vital than that of men. If we don't struggle to achieve equality in the sexual sphere, it is possible that achieving equity everywhere else will rest upon a shaky foundation. In other words, anatomy is not destiny so much as the social construction of anatomy is destiny.

HAS ANYONE SEEN THE WORM?

Laqueur ended his investigation with the publication of Freud's *Three Essays* in 1905. But the mystery doesn't end there. Lisa Jean Moore and Adele E. Clarke, two sociologists at San Francisco State University, picked up the trail of the ever-vanishing clitoris. In a wide-ranging analysis of twentieth-century medical literature, Moore and Clarke documented the deterioration of accuracy and detail in medical illustrations of the clitoris under the Freudian model.[28] They discovered that "the online University of California Melvyl Library Catalog found three records of books on the clitoris and 35 on the penis; a Current Contents title words search found 19 citations on the clitoris and 347 on the penis; and a Medline search found 78 articles with clitoris the keyword, and 1,611 with penis."

In examining anatomical representations of the clitoris, Moore and Clarke found that clitoral images in the first half of the twentieth century "varied from simple to complex," with a more generous supply of simple renderings. "Anatomies matter," they conclude, because they "create shared images which become key elements in repertories of bodily understanding touted around by all those who have seen them."

As mid-century approached, the work of Dr. Robert Latou Dickinson, a New York City gynecologist who was also a self-taught artist, provided an exception to these bland renditions. In his 1949 classic *Human Sex Anatomy: A Topographical Hand Atlas* he recorded the enormous normal variations in the appearance of women's genitalia, and illuminated the hidden parts beneath the surface of the skin.[29]

Despite Dickinson's widely known work, things deteriorated even further during the 1950s and 1960s. Eight post-Dickinson texts surveyed from the 1950s and 1960s "varied little in their treatment of the clitoris; they omitted it." In one book, our sleuths found "a worm-like, unlabeled part of the body which we assume to be the clitoris." Shortly after reading the article, I picked up my well-thumbed 1981 edition of *Taber's Cyclopedic Medical Dictionary* and, looking at the illustration of the female reproductive system found a squiggly, unlabeled dotted line.[30] The worm! To Taber's credit, later editions do label the glans, and the eighteenth edition provides the only illustration of the female genitals—in color—to be found in any standard medical reference, although you will not find the complete clitoris identified as yet.

Moore and Clarke did not include Masters and Johnson's work in their survey, but I want to mention it here because their work was so profoundly influential for a quarter of a century. In a climate more receptive to the public discussion of sexuality, the 1960s publication of *Human Sexual Response* finally brought discussion of the clitoris to light.[31] Indeed, the "first couple" of sex theory and therapy devoted an entire chapter to it, calling it both "a receptor and transformer of sensual stimuli," as well as an "organ" and an "organ system." Yet in purporting to dispel certain "phallic fallacies," Masters and Johnson actually created a new vaginal fiction, the so-called "orgasmic platform" located in the "outer third of the vagina." What they are really describing here are clitoral structures, which surround the vaginal opening. Since they firmly believe that the vagina and not the clitoris is "the human female's primary means of sexual expression," they apparently needed to concoct something impressive-sounding to back up this assumption.

THE REDISCOVERY OF THE MISSING CLITORIS

Although Masters and Johnson allude to a "clitoral system," and point out a number of equivalent structures of the clitoris and the penis, they failed to grasp the significance of these correspondences. Dr. Mary Jane Sherfey argued that because women's genital anatomy is equivalent to men's, women's capacity for sexual response should also be equivalent. Using Masters and Johnson's anatomical description of the penis, Sherfey found the clitoris to be a powerful organ system in contrast to the commonly accepted view of it as a diminutive pea-sized outcropping on the female vulva. Using established embryological evidence she debunked the conventional idea that the clitoris is a miniature penis, arguing instead that the male and female genitals are equivalent structures that function in similar ways to produce sexual pleasure and orgasm. In fact, Sherfey believed women's capacity for sexual response was even more powerful than men's for three specific reasons. First, women have a greater blood supply to the pelvic region and genitals. Second, women have longer and stronger pelvic muscles—both of these conditions are necessary for the potential demands of childbirth. Lastly, women have the innate (though largely unacknowledged) capacity to experience multiple orgasm. "The popular idea that a woman should have one orgasm which should bring 'full satisfaction,' act as a strong sedative, and alleviate sexual tension for several days to come is simply fallacious," Sherfey declared.[32] "That the female could have the same orgasmic anatomy (all of which are female to begin with) and not be expected to use it simply defies the very nature of the biological properties of evolutionary and morphogenic [structural evolution of an organism] processes."

Today Sherfey has been largely ignored by feminist sexologists. Some perceive her work as too steeped in biology, and she has also been dismissed for being an early disciple of Masters and Johnson. Nonetheless, her study is startling in its prescience, and it is all the more impressive because she was working in the very belly of the Freudian beast during the 1960s, when the term "feminist psycho-analyst" was considered an oxymoron, and the dramatic gains of feminist activism were a decade away. From a close reading of Sherfey's work, it does not seem that she was trying to prove that women's sexuality is "better" than men's, or that she was implying that orgasm was the only goal of sexual activity. Her point, I believe, was that by having their sexuality defined through male standards, women have only the dimmest idea of what their sexuality really is and have little sense of their sexual power. Sherfey's book was published in 1972, and when the FFWHCs discovered it in 1975, it provided the basis for their more comprehensive and anatomically accurate redefinition of the clitoris.

The tenacious buttressing of traditional gender norms is no joke. Once, when Suzann Gage and I were presenting a poster session on the clitoris at the American Public Health Association, we were attacked by two Ivy League MDs who created a huge scene by loudly denouncing our interpretation. Naturally, a large crowd gathered. With fire in their eyes, they told us that our interpretation was WRONG, and that we had NO RIGHT to be disagreeing with experts in the field. There have been others who have disagreed or disbelieved, Masters and Johnson and some feminists among them.

When I discovered Laqueur's book, I was astounded to see that someone had actually undertaken the arduous job of sifting through a bewildering array of texts in many languages over the vast stretch of two millennia to track down the story of the missing clitoris. Laqueur's study affirmed the FFWHCs intuitive inclination to reject the grossly inaccurate two-sex version of genital anatomy. He also provided documentation for the anatomical correctness in the reconceptualized depiction of the clitoris, which was unavailable in modern anatomy books. Moore and Clark's study showed us why getting professional validation for the redefinition of the clitoris had been so hard.

It is really quite astonishing that a small group of women without medical degrees, a clue about the history of the missing clitoris, or the intention of making medical history, money, or fame, reconceptualized women's genital anatomy in a way that should be the envy of any up-and-coming anatomist. They were on such intimate terms with their own anatomy that Sherfey's description of the clitoris made sense. Due to their reverence for women's bodies, the women at FFWHCs were able to make a conceptual leap that most anatomists have yet to make.

FEMALE EJACULATION Fact or Fantasy? 3

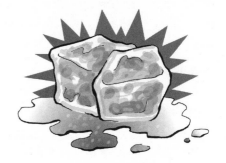

The idea that many women experience a spurt, gush, trickle, or dribble of clear, alkaline fluid during sexual response that is directly analogous to the fluid from the male prostate has been one of the most hotly debated questions in modern sexology. It is not, however, a new discussion. This phenomenon is mentioned in Chinese and Indian sex advice books as early as 500 B.C.E. Physicians and philosophers in ancient Greece were aware of the existence of glands around the female urethra that emit prostatic-like secretions, and such tissue was identified by anatomists during the Renaissance. Until the eighteenth century, when male and female sexuality began to be seen as radically different, there was no debate as to whether women "ejaculated," what caused it, or where the fluid came from. In the eighteenth and nineteenth centuries, the concept of female ejaculation was not discounted so much as obliterated due to the medical and social myopia through which women's sexuality was viewed. For the first eighty years of the twentieth century—with the exception of a few isolated journal articles by physicians interested in diseases of the female urethra—information about female ejaculation entirely disappeared from medical discourse, and from our concept of women's sexuality.

When Beverly Whipple and John Perry documented women's ability to ejaculate in the 1980s, it elicited a yawn from many sexologists, and disbelief and scorn from others. Many feminists were skeptical as well. Nevertheless, reliable studies have revealed that during intense sexual excitement, or as orgasm approaches, many women produce a clear, alkaline fluid that is *not* urine, which may vary in amount from a few drops to about a quarter of a cup (about two ounces), sometimes much more. Yet many women, and perhaps their partners as well, believe that this fluid is really urine. Whipple reports that some women find ejaculating this mysterious fluid embarrassing and suppress sexual response to avoid producing it. There are doctors who prescribe drugs to suppress the "urine," while others have performed surgeries to stop it.[33] Is it possible that these women are wetting the bed, dousing their partners, and splashing the walls with urine? Or are they experiencing a phenomenon analogous to male ejaculation?

Today, despite an impressive chain of historical evidence, several important contemporary studies, a tsunami of personal testimonies by women who experience ejaculation, and a collection of stunning visual images on video produced by feminist activists, most sexologists, physicians, and women themselves remain confused about female ejaculation. Even among the believers, there is still widespread disagreement as to how many women do ejaculate with regularity, why all women don't appear to ejaculate, and whether, as some proponents insist, it can be learned.

A FEMALE PROSTATE?

As we discovered in chapter 1, female genital tissue does not disappear after the seventh week of gestation (see page 32). As the fetus develops, testosterone kicks in for those with XY chromosomes. In order for men to develop a prostate gland, prostatic tissue must first exist in the female template. In the female embryo, the entire urethra and its surrounding tissue develops from the urogenital sinus, as does the portion of the male urethra that passes through the male prostate gland, called the prostatic urethra. The question we should be asking then, is not *if* a female prostate exists, not *if* women ejaculate, but how the female prostate differs from that of the male.

The male prostate gland is roughly the size and shape of a walnut, and it is located at the base of the bladder. The "prostatic" portion of the urethra passes through its core, and numerous small ducts connected to a labyrinthine system of tiny tubes inside the prostate open through two prostatic ducts into the urethral canal. The prostate gland produces a clear alkaline fluid, which, at orgasm, is squeezed out through the ducts into the urethra where it joins the sperm as it jets by. Men usually ejaculate from one-half to two ounces, and the secretions of the prostate make up about 15 percent of this amount.[34] Like the other seminal secretions, the prostate fluid is alkaline, which helps to keep the sperm alive in the vagina's acidic environment.

G SPOT OR URETHRAL SPONGE?

The concept of a hypersensitive area inside the vagina, the Grafenberg spot or "G spot," burst upon the world stage in 1981 with the publication of *The G Spot and Other Discoveries about Human Sexuality,* and has now become such an indelible cultural artifact that it has been awarded a spot in the dictionary.[35] In spite of its celebrity, there is still much confusion about what the G spot really is and where it is located, and many women are confused about whether or not they have one. These quandaries arose because the few researchers who have been interested in the issue chose to define it differently. Josephine Sevely and J. W. Bennett claimed that the tissue surrounding the female urethra was identical to the *corpus spongiosum* that surrounds the male urethra, and cited gynecologist John Huffman's study (see page 122) which shows up to thirty-one tiny prostatic-like glands embedded in it. Sevely simply referred to this tissue as "*corpus spongiosum*," as the corresponding tissue in the male is called.[36] This material was published in an expanded form in Sevely's book *Eve's Secrets: A New Theory of Female Sexuality*.[37]

In 1981, Beverly Whipple and John Perry published an article in the *Journal of Sex Research*, and named it the "Grafenberg spot," or the G spot.[38] In *A New View of a Woman's Body*, the FFWHCs included an unnamed structure surrounding the urethra in their comprehensive definition of the clitoris and called it the urethral sponge. Two illustrations show a woman placing a finger inside of her vagina and feeling the sponge. "In addition to ejaculation, some self-helpers have said that stimulation of the urethral sponge can be a focal point for sexual arousal and orgasm," the group noted. So *corpus spongiosum*, G spot, and the urethral sponge are all the same thing. Sevely's findings were published first, and her investigation was the most thorough and wide-ranging of the three. Whipple and Perry focused on the function of the G spot, linking stimulation of this spot to female ejaculation and orgasm, and they provided a wealth of personal accounts of women and their partners who had experienced or witnessed female ejaculation. Alice Kahn Ladas's suggestion that they write a popular book put the concept on the map in a way that endless articles in sexology journals could never have done. In the book, they write, "the Grafenberg Spot lies directly behind the pubic bone within the front wall of the vagina. It is usually located about halfway between the back of the pubic bone and the cervix, along the course of the urethra…. The size and exact location vary."[39] This description proved to be confusing for many women who couldn't find such a hypersensitive spot. Women who did not have orgasms through vaginal stimulation with fingers or the penis thought that they must not have a G spot. Originally, Whipple and Perry believed that stimulation of the G spot and female ejaculation resulted in orgasm, but Whipple later rejected this notion, noting that it might just increase pleasurable sensations. It seems that the FFWHCs' detailed description of the urethral sponge and their inclusion of it in their definition of the clitoris provide the clearest picture of the structure and how it fits into the larger clitoral system. It makes clear that the sponge is not a part of the vagina, although it may be bonded to the vaginal "roof" in some way. Their illustrations show exactly how to find the urethral sponge, and, most importantly, they make it clear that *every woman has one*. How sensitive the sponge, or a spot on it, may be varies from woman to woman.

IS IT URINE?

One of the reasons that female ejaculation has remained so controversial is that definitive studies on the fluid's constituents have never been done. In the early 1980s, Whipple and Perry found that prostatic acid phosphatase (PAP), an enzyme that is present in male prostatic secretions, and glucose (a sugar) were "substantially higher in the ejaculatory fluid [of women] than in the urine samples." Urea and creatinine, two of the principle constituents of urine, were "substantially lower in the ejaculatory than in the urine specimens."[40] This analysis suggests that female ejaculate is not urine.

In an effort to show that female ejaculate is not from the bladder, Edwin Belzer, who taught human sexuality courses at Dalhousie University in Nova Scotia, reported an interesting experiment done by one of his students who ejaculated easily. She took Urised—a bladder relaxant drug that turns the urine bright blue—several times during masturbation. Afterward, she found either a faint bluish tinge or no color on her sheets where she ejaculated. She then urinated on the sheet. That spot was a deep blue, indicating that there was plenty of blue dye in the urine, where it was supposed to be, but little or none in the ejaculate, where it was not supposed to be.[41]

The most recent study on female ejaculation, conducted by two Spanish researchers, Francisco Cabello Santamaria, a physicist and psychologist, and Rico Nesters, a clinical analyst, was reported at the Thirteenth World Congress of Sexology in Valencia, Spain, in 1997.[42] These researchers analyzed the urine of twenty-four women before and after orgasm for signs of prostatic secretions. Six of the women ejaculated and that, too, was analyzed. All of the women masturbated to orgasm and had not had sexual contact for two days. Their analysis focused on identifying the presence of prostate-specific antigen (PSA), since this is a primary chemical in male prostatic emissions.

The results of the Spanish study are impressive. In all cases, the preorgasmic urine was just that—urine. But PSA was present in 75 percent of the postorgasmic urine samples, and in all of the ejaculation samples. As expected, the amount of PSA was high in the ejaculation samples and lower in the postorgasmic urine. Cabello Santamaria surmised that the PSA is pushed into the bladder either because the sphincter muscle that holds in urine is weak, or because it opened momentarily during orgasm. (This phenomenon occurs in men who have had prostate surgery. It is called "retrograde [backward] ejaculation." Men who seek to delay ejaculation by squeezing the base of the penis (see page 169) may also experience this phenomenon.)

There may be another reason, however, that some women's postorgasmic urine contains PSA. Some of the glands may empty into the urethra, and if the ejaculate does not squirt out, it would remain in the urethra to be picked up by the first post-ejaculatory flow of urine.

Santamaria and Nesters express the hope that their investigation will have "a tranquilizing effect on women," first, to assure them "that it is a perfectly normal and, probably, common phenomenon," and second, to help those who do not experience it avoid "an 'endless quest' for their ejaculation, because they probably do ejaculate, but in scarce quantities."

These reports strongly suggest that the fluid coming out of the female urethra during sexual response is not urine, but are problematic in that they each evaluated the female ejaculate for different constituents. Male ejaculate has been analyzed exhaustively, and volumes have been written about its makeup. At least nine different substances are present in male prostatic fluid, including PAP, PSA, and fructose. There is, however, one test—the sniff test—that anyone can do at home to determine whether they are ejaculating or urinating. After sex, sniff the wet spot on your sheets. If you have urinated, you will smell the unmistakable acrid odor.

HOW MUCH DO WOMEN EJACULATE?

There have been different estimates of how much fluid women ejaculate. Sevely found that "the amount of prostatic fluid released through the female urethra may be as much as 126 milliliters (about one quarter of a cup, or four ounces)."[43] A quarter of a standard eight-ounce cup is actually two ounces, so it is not clear which measurement Sevely actually means. In *The G Spot*, Whipple and Perry reported that the amount of female ejaculate varied from "a few drops to about a quarter of a teaspoon," although they acknowledged that the range could be as high as a cup (eight ounces) or more.[44] Desmond Heath, a New York psychiatrist who conducted an extensive inquiry into the subject of female ejaculation over several years, suggests that "the pararuethral glands of Skene are capable of producing and ejecting impulses, associated with sexual stimulation, a clear watery fluid [from] two openings either side of the urethral meatus at a rate of 30 to 50 ccs [7 to 15 ounces] in 30 to 50 seconds."[45] Cabello Santamaria and Nesters report that they collected "up to 16 ml," or about five and one-half ounces.

In my own queries to women who ejaculate, estimates vary widely from a few drops to repeated gushes that require a mop up. One interviewee, Jenna, unabashedly classifies herself as a "gusher":

I used to take a towel to bed, but the ejaculate would soak through four thick folds and then I could literally ring the towel out. Finally I got a lambskin mat, which doesn't allow the liquid to seep through, and it's washable. Still, I often have to mop the floor when I'm finished. I have developed the ability to manipulate myself to repeatedly release ejaculatory fluid, given enough engorgement of erectile tissues and state of arousal.

Danielle told me:

One lover I had didn't believe in ejaculation, even after she squirted a dime-sized puddle on the bathroom floor one night. We smelled it and it had a mild, undefinable odor, but she thought it was urine. Then once, when I was sort of curled up in her arms with my knees behind her shoulder—splat!—I ejaculated all over her face and arms—I don't recall it as an orgasm necessarily, just very intense pleasure. After we recovered from our surprise, we evaluated it and decided that it would fill at least one standard test tube and about half of another [about an ounce and a half]. At that point, she changed her mind.

How can we account for the enormous variation in the amount of ejaculate? As noted on page 94, we know that the amount of male ejaculate ranges quite a bit, from one half to two ounces, and that the fluid produced by the prostate is about 15-20 percent of this, so there is some variation in the amount of prostatic fluid that men produce. It is clear, however, that many women produce much, much more.

Although there has yet to be a study of the effect that varying testosterone levels in women (or in men for that matter) may have on the production of prostatic fluid, it would seem that the amount of testosterone a woman has may be a determinant in how much ejaculate a woman produces. All women have some testosterone, and while the amount may be influenced by some lifestyle and environmental factors, genetic inheritance may be the strongest single factor.

There may be a number of reasons for the huge differential in the amounts of female ejaculate. Some women may simply have more, or bigger, glands than others, or their glands may normally produce more fluid, the way some people sweat much more than others. Some women who have had vaginal births may have weak or damaged pelvic floor muscles, and simply cannot get a strong squeeze from the muscles, while other women's glands may have been damaged or scarred from past infections so that the fluid doesn't come out, save for a drop or two from the glands that empty directly into the urethra. Other women may not ejaculate because their urethral glands have gotten lazy from a long-term lack of sexual activity or from the low intensity of their sexual response. Unknown hormonal factors may also suppress the production of prostatic fluid.

The world is divided into two groups when it comes to female ejaculation: those who believe that it exists, and those who don't. Most likely, those who ejaculate or have had a partner who does tend to be the believers, and those who do not see an obvious squirt from themselves or their partners are often the disbelievers. The Spanish study suggests that all women ejaculate, but that it ranges from too little to be noticed to the very obvious, and that in some women, it may be squeezed back into the bladder to emerge with the next urination.

Sevely suggested that one of the reasons many women do not think they ejaculate is that during intercourse, the urethral meatus, or opening, "is pushed inside the vagina" so that "if a woman ejaculates fluid only during coitus, the outlet of the fluid is obscured inside the vagina."[46] Even if the urethral opening is not pushed or pulled inside of the vagina, a woman's ejaculation is blocked by the penis or pubic mound. In this case, it ends up as a wet spot, which for some women is quite large.

Another reason many women do not appear to ejaculate is that their partner has his or her orgasm before she is fully sexually aroused, so the opportunity simply never arises. Women who have had urethritis, an infection of the urethra caused by gonorrhea or other bacteria, may have scarring along the urethra; the tiny paraurethral ducts may scar over, preventing ejaculation. Perhaps some older women, like older men, have decreased erectile and ejaculatory capability because of atherosclerosis—hardening of the arteries, which may affect ejaculatory capability. In *The G Spot*, and in early papers coauthored by Whipple and Perry, female ejaculation was closely linked to stimulation of the G spot, although it is noted that "a few women report that they also ejaculate through clitoral stimulation alone."[47] I've talked to many women who ejaculate and say that they have done so without putting so much as a finger in the vagina. Is vaginal stimulation necessary for female ejaculation? Once and for all, the answer is NO!

Can women *learn* to ejaculate? Some activists who are promoting education about female ejaculation believe that women can learn. Several women have told me that they "learned" to ejaculate after watching videos about it and strengthening their pelvic floor muscles. Certainly women can learn to *recognize* ejaculate that dribbles or oozes out, rather then squirts or gushes. It's quite possible that some women who suddenly "learn" to ejaculate may be getting more sexually aroused than usual by masturbating with unusual zest and are finally producing enough ejaculate to be noticeable. One can certainly learn to have multiple orgasms and perhaps some women may discover an ability to ejaculate when they become multiorgasmic.

VOICES OF EXPERIENCE

At least part of the reason that female ejaculation has not been more widely recognized is that women typically do not share their sexual experiences with each other. Men may discuss their experiences with each other more readily, but may be less willing to discuss their partners' ejaculatory ability, perhaps because they don't like women competing on what has historically been male turf. In speaking to groups of women about sexuality over the years, many have shared their experiences about female ejaculation. Often after one woman tells her story, others may recognize for the first time that they too ejaculate. It's not uncommon to hear laughter and a sigh of relief, and then an admission that "all this time I thought I was wetting the bed!" or "I always attributed the wet spot to my partner." Their testimonies always make others in the group understand that their experience is entirely normal.

Mikki learned about female ejaculation when she worked at one of the FFWHCs, and says that this information was enormously liberating:

I've got a long list of things to thank the feminist health movement for, but high on the list is knowing about female ejaculation. During sex, I worried and got embarrassed about the mess I seemed to make. Until I learned about the full anatomy of the clitoris and that other women had actually ejaculated, I held back during sex (with both women and men)—I had learned my lessons about wetting the bed. Now, I have a couple of plastic-backed pieces of fabric (3 feet by 5 feet works well for me) for no muss, no fuss. I put down my soak piece, and then we get it on and I can let go and shoot as much as I feel like. When I ejaculate I usually need inside stimulation of my spongy stuff (that's the urethral sponge of the clitoris). Two or three fingers are good for me. I have never tried to collect what I shoot out, but I have watched in amazement with my lover(s)—once it went in an arc about a foot high and landed about 2 feet away. It can be a little or it can be a lot (I guess a few tablespoons to a quarter cup). I don't ejaculate as much when I masturbate as when I have a partner. My ejaculate keeps me wet and helps me have more than one orgasm. It definitely isn't urine—doesn't smell like it or have the same color. It smells and tastes differently according to the time in my cycle and what I've eaten lately. My partner has said that it is either sort of sweet (around ovulation) or sort of metallic (closer to menses). I don't always ejaculate every time I make love, but now I know that I don't have to hold back. That's the main message to take from learning about female ejaculation: don't hold back, and at the risk of sounding clichéd, let it flow!

After many years of lying in the wet spot, Christie discovered that she was making it herself:

When I had sex exclusively with men, I noticed that after sex, there would be a huge cold wet spot on the bed—often as wide as eighteen inches, sometimes more. I naturally believed that it was all from the man, but that was before I knew how little many men actually ejaculate. When I started having sex with women and also began masturbating a lot, I still noticed the giant wet spot and began taking a towel to bed with me. A few times I've had what I consider very dramatic squirting episodes where the fluid hit my toes. Once when I was masturbating, it hit the sheet, which I was holding up with my left hand and fluid splashed back down on me. During these episodes, I seldom have anything in my vagina. It was usually from clitoral stimulation alone and the gush usually came prior to orgasm.

My friend Rose gave me an account that she and her lover Ocha wrote about her experiences with ejaculation. Here is an abbreviated version of their piece:

> I'd been working on my vaginal muscles for about a year before I saw a video of women discussing their personal experiences with ejaculation. I first ejaculated after my lover and I watched a video about female ejaculation together. Once we were sitting in chairs facing each other a few feet apart as we masturbated, and suddenly I began to ejaculate all over him for about 30 to 40 seconds. I don't ejaculate every time but I often do, and the amount varies quite a bit, and sometimes I do it without even having an orgasm.... According to Ocha, "It's not a competition, nor should there be any pressure to out-shoot anybody. It's just another delicious, wet, beautiful thing that women can do."[48]

Jenna, whose account of ejaculating large quantities of fluid appears on page 100, has thought a lot about the meaning of female ejaculation:

I'm very proud of my ability to ejaculate and enjoy celebrating it with someone who appreciates it. Yet I can choose not to do it. Some of my partners haven't liked it that I ejaculate so much, so if I don't trust them to be comfortable with it, I won't do it. I must say that my ejaculatory orgasms feel different than the non-ejaculatory ones. My pulse gets much higher and my vagina vibrates.

SEEING IS BELIEVING

For those who are still doubtful about female ejaculation, there are a handful of sexy, illuminating videos made by activists, which document some spectacular instances. Each one has its strengths, and all offer complementary information on how different women feel about and experience ejaculation.

The first video was produced by Beverly Whipple, who is, without a doubt, the modern godmother of female ejaculation. Because of the potentially sensational nature of the subject matter, Whipple took pains to make *Orgasmic Expulsions of Fluid in the Sexually Stimulated Female* as medical as possible. In this brief seven-minute video, we see two volunteers from the waist down, feet in stirrups, with a male doctor's gloved finger stimulating them vaginally. The video is designed to reassure women, and perhaps their doctors, that ejaculation is entirely normal. Even in the sanitized setting, the ejaculations are quite impressive.

One of the messages of this video, which Whipple has since revised, is that stimulation of the G spot is the route to female ejaculation. We now know that vaginal stimulation of the G spot on the urethral sponge may or may not result in ejaculation and orgasm.

Dorrie Lane, a San Francisco sexuality educator, made *The Magic of Female Ejaculation*, the first nonmedical video on the subject. Dorrie provides some history of female ejaculation, an anatomy lesson, and supportive information in an upbeat, down-to-earth manner. She talks about how she first ejaculated and demonstrates how she does it. During the ejaculation segment, you can clearly see the tip of Dorrie's urethral sponge peeping through the vaginal opening.

Fanny Fatale, a sex educator and producer of erotic videos, made *How to Female Ejaculate*. Fanny takes time to include essential information about the anatomy of the clitoris and urethral sponge, then she and three friends, including champion ejaculator Shannon Bell (see below), discuss their experiences with each other and demonstrate how it happens for them. Carol Queen, author of *Exhibitionism for the Shy* (see Resources) says that she ejaculated for years before she knew what was really happening and that it makes her angry that she "had to struggle [to understand] something that's my birthright."

Carol observes that her ejaculate tastes salty and briny, like buttered popcorn, or like the floor of the forest. Fanny says that hers hardly has any smell.

Even though all four women ejaculate often, the difference in their experiences are remarkable. And, if you want to see part of the urethral sponge, here's your chance: Fanny's can be seen clearly just inside of her vaginal opening as she masturbates.

Nice Girls Don't Do It is a short video produced by Kathy Daymond, starring Shannon Bell, a woman renowned for her ability to ejaculate on a dime. While she ejaculates any number of times, Shannon provides information about anatomy, and discusses the role ejaculation has in her sexuality. Unfortunately the voiceover on the soundtrack competes with coffee-shop chatter in the background, which is intended to provide a casual air to something potentially shocking, but the din becomes intensely cloying, disrupting the viewer's concentration. Nonetheless the visual images are impressive, and Shannon has a compelling philosophical take on the subject.

Female ejaculation is just one of the topics addressed in *The Sluts and Goddesses Video Workshop, or How to Be a Sex Goddess in 101 Easy Steps*, by Annie Sprinkle and Maria Beatty. The intent of this imaginative and entertaining video encourages women to discover the power, intensity, and variety of sexual experience. In the first part, Annie and her friends explore their interest in dressing up, being sexy, and having fun with sex. Annie then discusses female ejaculation, demonstrating her own technique, which brings her to a five-minute orgasm that is not to be missed.

I highly recommend these videos to anyone who wants see some super-ejaculators in action. Many women have told me that after seeing one or more of the videos, they finally understood how it all happens. My friend Eileen, who had never ejaculated, called me from California one day out of the blue.

"I just had to tell you that I ejaculated!" she exclaimed.

"How did it happen?" I asked.

"My boyfriend and I were watching a video on female ejaculation, and we were fooling around for a couple of hours, and suddenly, it just happened. Boom! Ejaculation!"

Was she more turned on than usual?

"Yeah," she said, "I think it was the idea that I could ejaculate that got me so turned on."

These videos are listed in Resources on page 228.

WHY ARE PEOPLE OPPOSED TO FEMALE EJACULATION?

While female ejaculation has been discussed for most of recorded history throughout a variety of cultures, it remains a controversial issue. Although Whipple and Perry's study of the content of women's ejaculate has been widely criticized, there has yet to be a definitive study. The Spanish study mentioned on page 97 is a start, but it has not been published in a mainstream sexology journal. The videos that have been done also confirm that women can ejaculate, but some critics, including Beverly Whipple, believe that some of the women in these videos are only squirting diluted urine.[49]

Perhaps another reason for the slow acceptance of female ejaculation that superstar sexologists such as Kinsey, and Masters and Johnson, did not believe that some women ejaculate, in direct contradiction to their own observations. Kinsey and his colleagues denied that women ejaculated, although they observed that "muscular contractions of the vagina following orgasm may squeeze out some of the genital secretions, and in a few cases eject them with some force."[50] Masters and Johnson likewise deny that female ejaculation occurs. "Despite a popular misconception, most women do not ejaculate during orgasm," they insist. Their proof? "The erroneous belief that women ejaculate probably stems from descriptions in erotic novels of fluid gushing from the vagina as a woman writhes and moans at the peak moment of sexual passion." Yet they note that fourteen of the three hundred women in their own studies described a "gushing or expulsion of fluid at orgasm." They also admit that "we *have* [emphasis in original] observed several cases of women who expelled a type of fluid that was not urine."[51]

After an exhaustive quest to find a medical explanation for the copious ejaculations of a patient, Desmond Heath, an attending physician in psychiatry at New York City's Mount Sinai Hospital, came up dry. In desperation, he called the Masters and Johnson Institute, and reached the master himself. "Five minutes on the phone with Masters convinced me that the knowledge [of female ejaculation] had never been lost for it had never been known."[52]

Many sexologists who are typically somewhat sympathetic to women's issues refuse to accept the existence of female ejaculation, demanding more rigorous standards of proof. Likely they will sit comfortably in their disbelief, because there is zero scientific funding for studies on women's sexuality, unless it is on sexual *dys*function, and it is rare that researchers can support such studies on their own. Until the time when funding becomes available, we will just have to take women's word on ejaculation and await the science to confirm their testimonies.

In an article in *On Our Backs*, the renowned feminist sexzine, Fanny Fatale suggests one reason for the lack of acceptance of this phenomenon: "Society cannot accept female ejaculation precisely because it makes men and women equal."[53]

WHAT'S THE POINT?

Some women may find the idea of having a prostate gland—or many prostate glands—preposterous or don't like to think that they have a sexual structure that is so quintessentially masculine. Others may not like the idea because ejaculation is so firmly associated with the performance aspects of men's sexuality. Some feminist commentators are also concerned that if we incorporate female ejaculation into our concept of women's sexuality, it will become some sort of standard for "great sex," and that women who do not have spectacular ejaculations like the ones shown in videos will feel inadequate. These are serious and legitimate concerns, especially in light of the trend to downplay the "performance" aspects of sex. Regardless of how many women ejaculate, they should have access to detailed information about it. Just knowing that ejaculation is a normal part of women's sexuality can help us see it for what it really is—an expression of intense sexual pleasure. Knowing precisely where the fluid comes from can dispel shame or fear of "wetting the bed," and can further prevent many women from suppressing their sexual response to avoid it. It may also help others avoid undergoing disfiguring medical procedures to "fix" it. Whether or not we all ejaculate, just knowing that many of us do can help us to see our sexuality as more active, assertive, and powerful than we had previously believed.

THE MEDICALIZATION OF THE FEMALE PROSTATE

Leonore Tiefer, who is leading the movement against the medicalization of sexuality, is concerned that given "the insatiability of the media for the commercial potential of sexual topics," the possibility of female ejaculation would result in yet another performance standard for women to meet. Tiefer is also concerned that women who cannot find a G spot or do not have visible ejaculation will feel compelled to consult a sex therapist, and "that's not the most empowering message" we should be giving to women.[54]

Like most doctors, urologists, whose work focuses on the male prostate gland and erectile dysfunction, have ignored the female prostate and its role in sexual response. Yet, some critics have proposed that urological neglect may not be all that bad. In a contemporary critique of Huffman's paper (see page 122), a colleague wrote:

I rather wish that Dr. Huffman had not found it so convenient to apply the term female prostate to the group of glands under consideration. This is not a new concept, and this anatomical concept in the past has led, upon the part of certain eminent urologists, to an overly enthusiastic adoption of the clinical concept of female prostatism. This idea has resulted in the too frequent use of the cautery punch [destruction of tissue by burning as with a tiny hot poker or electric probe], or resectoscope [surgical removal using telescope-like instrument for visualization] on the female vesical orifice…

Furthermore, I am convinced that the use of the cautery punch or resectoscope on the vesical neck [part of the urethra attached to the bladder] of the female carries with it certain dangers of intractable sphincter incompetence [inability to hold urine] or even vesicovaginal fistula [formation of a pocket in the urethral wall in which urine becomes trapped].[55]

This is no idle fantasy. The above-mentioned treatments, along with others such as urethral dilation, are routinely employed by urologists today as a treatment for chronic urinary urgency and frequency, referred to as lower urinary tract sensitivity (LUTS). These treatments are often performed when there are no specific causes for the symptoms, although no well-designed studies document their usefulness.

Nonetheless, Ruben Gittes and Robert Nakamura, urologists at the Scripps Clinic and Research Foundation in California, note the increasing acceptance of the concept of a female prostate among urologists: "In the past decade, the availability of the specific histochemical staining for prostate-specific antigen (PSA) has rehabilitated the status of the paraurethral glands and spotlighted them as the homologue of the prostate." Like Huffman, Gittes and Nakamura are only concerned with female prostate diseases, not the sexual function. In fact, Gittes says he believes that there is *no* ejaculatory potential in women.[56]

These are serious issues that must be addressed in a thoughtful and responsible manner. Research should focus on understanding and explaining female ejaculation. Doctors should make genuine efforts to acquaint themselves with the sexual function of the female prostate to avoid treating a perfectly normal sexual function. We can hope (I know that I am dreaming) that the media will avoid the temptation to sensationalize female ejaculation, and instead concentrate on educating the public about it in conjunction with a genuine exploration of women's sexuality.

THE LOST HISTORY OF FEMALE EJACULATION

The earliest mention of female ejaculation appears in one of the first Chinese sex advice books, *Secret Methods of the Plain Girl*, a compendium of sexual practices from the time of the Yellow Emperor, the first emperor of China: "Her Jade Gate [vagina], becomes moist and slippery; then the man should plunge into her very deeply. Finally, copious emissions from her Inner Heart begin to exude outward."[57] In this context, "plain" may actually mean "pure" rather than unattractive or boring, while "inner heart" is clearly not the heart that pumps blood, but a colorful metaphor for the female prostate.

The Kama Sutra of Vatsyayana, the famous ancient Indian sexuality advice book, observes that "the semen of women continues to fall from the beginning of the sexual union to its end, in the same way as that of the male," indicating the copiousness of female ejaculate, and suggesting that women's ejaculate squirts or "falls" as a man's does.[58]

Although the Greeks didn't understand precisely how conception occurred, they were intensely curious about it, and believed that fertilization was somehow due to sexual secretions. A reference to what is clearly female ejaculation appears in the works of a disciple of the Greek physician Hippocrates. During the time of conception, he writes, "if the ejaculate of the man runs together directly with that from the woman, she will conceive."[59] Here, the word "ejaculate" seems to mean exactly that, and not the less concentrated effluent which we know as "vaginal sweating," or the few drops of viscous mucous secretion from the vulvovaginal glands (see page 46).

Aristotle had a somewhat muddled view of reproduction. He believed that conception was caused by elements contained in the male ejaculate, and that female fluids only contributed to nurturing the fetus. Yet, when he discussed women's genital anatomy, he produced a marvelously intuitive description of the anatomical mechanism by which women ejaculate:

> The path along which the semen passes in women is of the following nature: they possess a tube—like the penis of the male, but inside the body—and they breathe through this by a small duct which is placed above the place through which women urinate. This is why, when they are eager to make love, this place is not in the same state as it was before they were excited.[60]

It would seem that Aristotle is distinguishing between the female urethra, which is just inside the body, and the male urethra, much of which is located externally. The "small duct" could only be one of the paraurethral ducts, located beside or, as he notes, "above" the urethral opening. The claim that women also breathe through these ducts is ambiguous, but probably derives from Greek notions about how body fluids are produced. In the last sentence Aristotle notes the changes in "this place," the area surrounding the urethra during sexual excitement. He may be implying that the urethral sponge becomes larger and erect when women are sexually aroused. In the second century C. E., Galen asserted that women had testicles (ovaries) and of course, elaculated.[61]

There seems to have been no question about the existence of female ejaculation in the seventeenth century. The English physician Laevinius Lemnius observed that a woman "draws forth the man's seed, and casts her own with it" and "takes more delight, and is more recreated by it."[62] The French obstetrician Francois Mauriceau found that "the glands near [the urethra's] outer end are relevant to sexual pleasure because they pour out great quantities of saline liquor during coition, which increases the heat and enjoyment of women."[63] Danish gynecologist Kaspar Bartholin's description of the vagina directly echoes that of Aristotle and Galen when he renders a portrait of what can only be the urethral sponge. It "becomes longer or shorter, broader or narrower, and swells sundry ways according to the lust of the woman," Bartholin explained. This structure is "of a hard and nervous flesh, and somewhat spongy, like the Yard." ("Yard" is a measurement term used in Renaissance England to describe the penis.)

Bartholin's observation is remarkably easy to verify. If you (or your partner) insert a finger into the vagina before sexual response and press toward the pubic mound, you will feel the moist, ridged walls of the vagina—nothing more. Do the same thing during sexual response and press upward, you will feel a dramatic change. The sponge may feel different in different women, as Bartholin noted, "longer or shorter, broader or narrower," and may swell in various ways, depending perhaps on how excited a woman is. During the seventeenth century "nervous" meant "strong" or "vigorous," rather than "highly excitable," "unnaturally uneasy," or "apprehensive," as it does today. Thus, Bartholin's characterization of the clitoral sponge as "of a hard and nervous flesh" vividly renders it similar to the penile sponge: firm and vigorous. If we fast-forward to the present, the videos on female ejaculation, reviewed on pages 108–111, show the tip of the sponge protruding underneath the skin around the urethra, and sometimes it can be seen actually protruding through the vaginal opening.

In 1672, the renowned Dutch embryologist Regnier de Graaf published the results of an intensive investigation of women's "generative organs," including meticulous dissection and illustration of the tissue surrounding the female urethra. Citing Galen and Herophilus, another well-known Greek physician, as authorities on the subject, de Graaf describes "a whitish, membranous substance about one finger breadth thick which completely surrounds the urethral canal… [that] could be called quite aptly the female prostate." De Graaf goes on to say that "the function of the 'prostate' is to generate a pituito-serous juice [mucus mixed with a clear watery fluid] which makes women more libidinous with its pungency and saltiness and lubricates their sexual parts in agreeable fashion during coitus."[64]

In the 1880s, the American gynecologist Alexander J. C. Skene also conducted an investigation into the makeup of the female prostate.[65] In a report of over a hundred dissections and several cases of chronic urethral infection, Skene identified two tiny ducts on either side of the urethra leading to two glands embedded in the surrounding spongy tissue. He succeeded in getting these two glands named after himself, but his inquiry only scratched the surface. Had Skene and his successors been aware of the historical record, they might have discovered (or *re*discovered, as it were) several dozen additional glands deeper inside of the urethral sponge that feed into the two large paraurethral glands. A few of the glands, called periurethral glands, open directly into the urethra.[66]

In one of the most widely read sex advice books (or "marriage manual" as such books were billed in the past), *Ideal Marriage: Its*

Physiology and Technique, published in successive editions from 1928 through the 1950s, the Dutch sexologist Theodore H. van de Velde addressed the issue of female ejaculation:

> So far as I can form an opinion on this subject, it appears that the majority of laymen believe that something is forcibly squirted (or propelled or extruded), or expelled from the woman's body in orgasm, and should so happen normally, as in the man's case. Finally it is at least just as certain that such an 'ejaculation' does not take place in many women of sexually normal functions, as that it does take place in others.[67]

Van de Velde's report appears to be based on the personal ejaculation accounts of his patients since he notes that "laymen" believe that it occurs. His speculation that ejaculation does not occur in many women may be incorrect, although it was probably a reasonable assessment, since many women either may not have recognized it or produced enough fluid to be noticed.

The classic modern study of the female prostate was performed by John W. Huffman, a gynecologist at Chicago's Northwestern University Medical School. In his 1948 article, Huffman provides a summary of medical citations on the subject, starting with Galen, through the 1930s. The article also contains intricate drawings of the tissue surrounding the urethra made from laboriously constructed wax models of urethras obtained from eleven different cadavers. Huffman exposes Skene's error in identifying only two ducts and glands near the urethral opening. One of his models shows up to thirty-one glands embedded in the labyrinthine erectile tissue surrounding the urethra. Cross sections of these models and several accompanying photos taken through a microscope show the distribution of the glands throughout the urethra, with the densest concentration in the middle section. The largest ones (those that Skene identified) are situated closer to the urethral opening. Describing the female prostate, Huffman commented, "The urethra might well be compared to a tree about which and growing outward from its base are numerous stunted branches, the paraurethral ducts and glands."[68]

Although the sole and only function of any gland is to manufacture and secrete a particular type of substance, Huffman, Skene, and other modern researchers were only interested in the disease potential of the paraurethral glands.

Dr. Ernest Grafenberg, a German gynecologist who immigrated to New York City before World War II, was the first modern sex researcher to take an interest in the secretions of the female prostate, and their role in women's sexuality. Having observed women masturbating to orgasm in a clinical setting, Grafenberg asserted that "one can see that large quantities of a clear, transparent fluid are expelled not from the vulva, but out of the urethra in gushes." He also makes the astute observation that "the profuse secretions coming out with the orgasm have no lubricating significance, otherwise they would be produced at the beginning of intercourse and not at the peak of orgasm."[69]

In spite of the recognition of a female prostate and its specific role in women's sexual response throughout history, Huffman's work on its structure and Grafenberg's attempt to explain its sexual function had little impact. The urethral sponge and the glands that it contains remained anatomical curiosities until the early 1980s, when several sexuality researchers, such as Beverly Whipple and John Perry, focused attention on them and named the part of the urethral sponge that can be felt through the vaginal wall the "G spot."

RECLAIMING THE FEMALE PROSTATE

In the mid-1970s, Josephine Lowndes Sevely, a Harvard graduate student in psychology, undertook a study of female ejaculation. In the introduction to her book *Eve's Secrets: A New Theory of Female Sexuality*, Sevely says that she had come across numerous references to "female fluids" and was aware of "the open acceptance of the phenomenon in other cultures in earlier times when awareness of 'female semen,' ...was a part of scientific and popular belief."[70] Sevely conducted an intensive search of historical, medical, and anthropological literature and found a wealth of references. *Eve's Secrets* documents the widespread acceptance of the phenomenon through the ages and includes a revealing survey of non-Western cultures as well, ranging from ancient Greek and Judaic texts to modern anthropological accounts of Native American and Pacific Islands cultures.

Whipple became interested in female ejaculation in the late 1970s when she was treating women with stress urinary incontinence (SUI). One of her clients with very strong pelvic floor muscles complained that she typically lost urine only during sex. "This just didn't make any sense to me," Whipple says. "Women with strong pelvic floor muscles aren't likely to suffer from incontinence."[71]

Whipple teamed up with John Perry and opened up the subject of female ejaculation to public scrutiny and discussion. A chapter on the subject was included in *The G Spot and Other Recent Discoveries about Human Sexuality*, cowritten with Alice Kahn Ladas, a well-known bioenergetic analyst and sex therapist.[72] (See pages 94–96 for a discussion of the G spot.) "I thought it extremely important to validate the sexual experiences that may vary from accepted norms," explains Whipple. "I also wanted to help women avoid surgery for SUI when they really didn't have it."[73]

In addition to including a chapter on female ejaculation in *The G Spot*, Whipple published articles and lectured at conferences on the subject, and even made a film showing women ejaculating in a clinical setting (see page 108), but many sexologists remain unconvinced. In that vacuum, feminists interested in sexuality began to share their own experiences, and several made videos (see pages 109–111).

After a flurry of interest from a handful of researchers in the 1980s, few medical studies have looked at urethral anatomy or female ejaculation. A 1998 Australian study published in the prestigious *Journal of Urology* conducted careful dissections of female cadavers and found that "current anatomical descriptions of female human urethral and genital anatomy are inaccurate" and that "end organ erectile tissue was surprisingly different from the descriptions of it in anatomy publications." The authors discovered that the urethra is attached to the vaginal wall, but "in all other directions it is surrounded by erectile tissue." Although these researchers did not look for prostate glands, they concluded that the sexual function of the urethra is an issue that should be investigated.[74]

Now we know that the existence of a female prostate and the phenomenon of female ejaculation are fact, not fantasy. We know that the amount of fluid produced varies greatly, from unnoticeable or a teaspoon or so to copious gushes. We know that ejaculation may occur with or without stimulation inside of the vagina and that it may accompany orgasm, or it may occur simply as a sign of intense sexual pleasure without orgasm. Even for women who regularly produce lots of fluid, orgasm may occur without ejaculation. There is just no set pattern. We do not know why some women ejaculate more than others. It is also unclear as to whether it can be "learned," although some women discover that they do ejaculate by enhancing their sexual response. Chapters 4 and 5 describe ways that women are exploring and expanding their sexual repertoires. Even if you don't discover an ability to ejaculate, you are likely to discover new and more rewarding ways of giving and receiving pleasure.

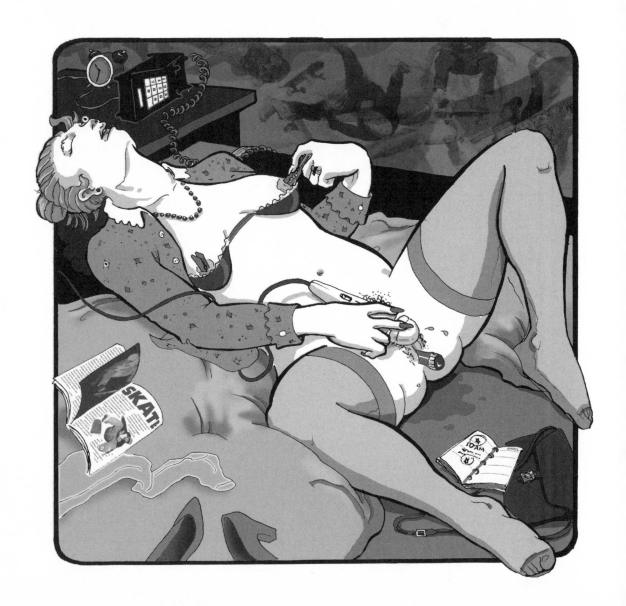

DOING IT FOR OURSELVES
Women Expand
Their Sexual Repertoire

4

S ex—how we think about it and how we do it—has changed more in the last three decades than it has in the last four or five thousand years, and it is exhilarating to think that these changes have primarily benefited women. Due to the mass marketing of the Pill, the wide availability of other types of contraception, and the legalization of abortion, for the first time in recorded history, women can have sex without fear of pregnancy and thus have a measure of sexual freedom that was previously unattainable. Feminists have led the struggle to rescue masturbation from antisex zealotry, claiming it as a technique for self-discovery and self-pleasuring, as well as for enriching partner sex. Many young women are refusing to be bound by rigid gender roles and some are even identifying themselves as bisexual rather than as exclusively heterosexual or lesbian. Tired of male-centered "fuck-'n'-cum" pornography, feminists are writing, filming, and performing and distributing their own postporn erotica. A few enterprising feminists have established boutiques and mail-order catalogs catering to women, making vibrators, sex toys, sex advice books, and erotica widely available. Others are offering workshops that help women break out of unrewarding sexual patterns and explore their sexuality and enhance their sexual response.

These are just some of the most visible changes that are beginning to transform the long-standing male-centered heterosexual model of sexuality. After thirty years of change and evolution, sex is definitely different for women in ways that our grandmothers could hardly have imagined.

IS IT SEX OR JUST FOOLIN' AROUND?

Perhaps the most important change now under way is the movement to redefine sex as far more than intercourse. This shift is occurring but remains a revolution in progress. President Clinton's repeated denial that he and Monica Lewinsky were having sex is just one of myriad examples of how far we still have to go. While many people clearly thought of their encounters as "sex," according to standard reference books, they were merely fooling around. *Sex in America: A Definitive Survey* finds that "vaginal intercourse is... what people imagine when they think of sex."[75] The streetwise, up-to-date *Random House Dictionary of the English Language* defines "to have sex" as "to engage in intercourse." The definition of "the sex act" in the authoritative *Complete Dictionary of Sexology (CDS)* is "a colloquial term for copulation, sexual intercourse, or coitus."[76]

President Clinton's definition was correct according to the prevailing notion, and the irony is that most if not all of the president's most vociferous critics probably believe that, too. My question is that if "fooling around" is so great as to cause the constitutional crisis of the century, why would anybody want to limit their physical interactions to intercourse?

This is not to say that intercourse isn't enjoyable. A number of women prefer it above any other form of sexual expression. "I just love the delicious sensations of penetration," Diane says. "Besides orgasm, it's my favorite part."

"I feel so full and connected to my partner during intercourse, and I almost always come that way," Jodie reports.

Many women, however, find lots of sexual benefits from non-intercourse sex. I was recently at a dinner party with a dozen or so women doctors. When the conversation turned to sex, one woman piped up, "I've been dating a seventy-two-year-old man. He can't get an erection, and, let me tell you, it's the best sex I've ever, *ever* had!"

"You go girl!" I thought, but I had the sense that her enthusiastic endorsement of the joys of non-intercourse sex met with skepticism among many at the table.

In a marvelously canny essay entitled "Are We Having Sex Now or What?," Greta Christina, one of the new "sexpert" generation who is actively exploring and critiquing contemporary sexual practices, personally assesses the question of sex.[77] She kept a list of the men with whom she had intercourse, but when she started having sex with women, she realized she needed a more inclusive definition, and then things got more complicated. "As I kept doing more kinds of sexual things, the line between *sex* and *non-sex* kept getting more hazy and indistinct," she writes. "I know when I'm feeling sexual...but feeling sexual with someone isn't the same as having sex with them... Even being sexual with someone isn't the same as *having* sex with them." Some of Christina's friends suggested, "If you thought of it as sex when you were doing it, then it was." Naturally, this brought up the issue of "what do I think it *is*?" She tried to construct a definition. "Perhaps having sex with someone is the conscious, consenting, mutually acknowledged pursuit of shared sexual pleasure," she thought. What if one or neither partner was able to derive pleasure? What if one person is asleep? "Can you have a situation where one person is having sex and the other isn't?" she asks. "It seems that no matter what definition I come up with, I can think of some real-life experience that calls it into question." What about S/M games without any genital contact? What about a sex worker who's turned on while a client watches her masturbate? Is that sex, or work for hire?

Christina provides a thought-provoking and very instructive inquiry. In the end, though, she doesn't come up with an entirely satisfactory definition, illustrating just how complex, nuanced, variously constructed, often vexing, and many-splendored sexual interactions can be.

REWRITING THE INTERCOURSE SCRIPT

The sexual script that most men learn in their youth is entirely goal oriented. The goal, of course, is to experience the maximum pleasure of an orgasm as quickly and efficiently as possible. The surreptitious masturbation that most boys engage in allows for a prolonged period of experimentation, in which they learn what is pleasurable and how to achieve it in as short a time and with as little effort as possible. In this context, goal orientation seems entirely reasonable. According to most reports, the average male orgasm occurs within two to five minutes after direct penile stimulation begins. If the goal is a single orgasm, and quality is of no concern, then this pattern works quite well for men.

As the Kinsey report notes, "Exceedingly few males modify their attitudes of sex or change their overt behavior in a fundamental way after their mid teens."[78] The problem is that when adolescent boys begin to have sex with girls or other boys, this well-rehearsed script is passed on whole cloth and becomes the template for girls' sexual scripts as well. Like the hand, the firm moist grip of the vagina provides the stimulation that is likely to result in male orgasm with as little effort as possible.

One of the most important changes that feminists have advocated is taking the focus off of intercourse and rewriting the sexual "script."

The notion that not every sexual encounter includes intercourse may come as a shock to many heterosexual men whose well-honed masturbation script is focused on the most efficient route to an orgasm. Even when men are considerate of their female partners' needs, once intercourse is initiated, it usually results in male orgasm. After that, even if a man is up for the job, as it were, his hormone levels drop precipitously, and subsequently his enthusiasm for continuing sex is considerably diminished.

It takes many women far longer than men to become fully aroused—as long as a half-hour in many cases. California sexologists William Hartman and Marilyn Fithian monitored over 20,000 orgasms and found that it takes an *average* of twenty minutes for women to reach orgasm in the laboratory. For many women, it can take up to a half-hour or more of sustained stimulation to move into orgasmic range.[79]

If orgasm is the goal, then moving the attention off of intercourse will equalize a woman's chances of achieving it. The key is for men to learn ejaculatory control. By varying the type and intensity of stimulation to the penis, men can learn to provide their partners with an equal chance to explore the peaks and valleys, and perhaps the hidden nooks and crannies of their sexual response. We'll look at the issue of male ejaculatory control in chapter 5.

For many years, sexologists and family planning advocates have been promoting the idea of "outercourse," a form of sexual activity that includes everything that partners find sexy and pleasurable *except* vaginal or anal intercourse. "Outercourse is the most exquisite way of experiencing sexual pleasure without exchanging bodily fluids," Whipple points out.[80] In the age of AIDS, the idea of women and men having rewarding sex without vaginal or anal penetration has taken on a heightened, sexuality-enhancing, and in some cases *lifesaving* significance. People who are disabled or seriously or chronically ill have long employed outercourse when intercourse is painful or impossible.

Many women, and surely some men as well, have mourned the loss of the heavy petting that was the sexual norm before the advent of the Pill and legal abortion. Petting allowed women to get as good as they gave, and to get it at great length. Since intercourse was less of an option, sex became a hothouse of desire to be explored and experienced at leisure.

Sunny recalls the spring of her junior year at college when she and her boyfriend had passionate outercourse in the bathtub. "We lived in a group house, and the bathroom was the only place we could have any privacy. It was a Catholic college, and the Student Health Service did not provide contraception, and I couldn't afford a private doctor. We would bathe each other, do soapy massages, style our hair with bubbles, and masturbate ourselves and each other." Sunny recalls the sex that she had in that tub as the best of her life. "It's just never been so inventive," she says wistfully.

Ruth, a sex therapist from California, relates her youthful experience with outercourse. "My boyfriend and I wanted to save intercourse for marriage, but that didn't stop us from having ecstatic sex. We explored ourselves and each other and learned how to fantasize and kiss and touch in very imaginative ways. When we were finished, we always felt like we'd been transported to hyperspace."

Rosalind, who has had many sexual experiences with both women and men, describes what she recalls as the most erotic night of her life. "At an office party, I started dancing with one of the executives I had a crush on, and it turned out to be mutual. He invited me to his place. We started talking about what we thought about each other, fantasies we'd had about each other, and that escalated into sex. I didn't have my cervical cap, and he had no condoms, so we did everything but intercourse over and over all night long. I was so dizzy that I would have an orgasm if he blew in my ear. Finally at dawn, we had to go sit in the bathtub to cool down and get our heads back together."

Many lesbians and bisexual women who come out after having sex exclusively with men say that sex with women opened up unimagined new worlds of pleasure.

My all-time-favorite piece of erotic literature is a wildly funny riff by Sdiane Bogus (a pseudonym) called "Dyke Hands," in which the narrator explores the ravishing sexual potential we hold in our fingertips:

> Because dyke hands are the sexual organs of lesbian love, they can be as shocking to view as the penis through an open fly, or as bold (delicious) to behold as the breast of a woman suddenly uncovered... [Those hands] belong to our lovers, and those very hands come to our beds outstretched to touch, to rub, to tickle, to smooth, to run ripples of pleasure over our bodies, and often we take those very hands, finger by precious finger, into our mouths, assuming their cleanliness, their sanctity, and perform fingerlingus.

The narrator and her lover go for a manicure, and the results are explosive.

> Massaging and drawing with a near-pornographic stroke, the manicurist pulled her own encircled hand down my lover's arm, smoothly, pressing with sensual surety every molecule of lotion into the pores of her hand and arm.... There were my lover's ten virile fingers stretched out like a naked man before

a geisha.... How good these hands were to my flesh when their touch wrought magic fires in my feet, raised the hair on my arms, brought my clitoris to knot and explosion.

In spite of her rapturous fantasy, the narrator suddenly has misgivings about the public display of hands that perform such intimate caresses.

The hands that stroke my hair, caress my flesh, that grip my thighs, press my love button, that slide between the satin readiness of my labia, ought not to be seen by the daily populace.... My holiest orgasms come from the probing phalanges of my lover's dyke hands. I'd not like to have them generally touching every Tom, Dick, and Harriet, not my dyke's hands.[81]

These accounts illustrate how extravagantly incendiary and exquisitely intimate non-intercourse sex can be, and, for those of us who have forgotten, they remind us that intercourse is only one way to experience the rich banquet of sexuality.

MASTURBATION
As Natural as Breathing?

Masturbation is as old as life itself. And, it appears to be innate. Gynecologists and ultrasound technicians are familiar with the sight of male fetuses with erect penises. A report from a group of Italian obstetricians published in the *American Journal of Obstetrics and Gynecology* describes similar activity of a female fetus during an ultrasound examination:

> We recently observed a female fetus at 32 weeks' gestation touching the vulva with fingers of [her] right hand. The caressing movement was centered primarily on the region of the clitoris. Movements stopped after 30 to 40 seconds, and started again after a few moments. Further, these light touches were repeated and were associated with short, rigid movements of the pelvis and legs. After another break, in addition to this behavior, the fetus contracted the muscles of the trunk and limbs, and the climax, clonicotonic movements [rapid muscle contractions] of the body, followed. Finally she relaxed and rested. We [several doctors and the mother] observed this behavior for about 20 minutes.[82]

Fetal masturbation? Female fetuses having orgasms? A resounding yes to both of these questions. This represents some very bad news for the antimasturbation lobby, since there are no pure foods, stern admonitions, or aluminum mittens that can prevent interuterine sex play. Babies as young as three or four months old have been reported to masturbate, and certainly many young children do.

Most people probably remember masturbating as children, but because it was done in secret, many assume that they were the only ones who did such a thing. Here are a few experiences that people have shared with me:

Marci remembers being enamored at age five by a *Life* magazine cover featuring a huddle of all-star football players. "I was awash with desire. I would sit and stare at that picture, touching myself lightly. I don't specifically remember having 'orgasms,' but these were intensely erotic experiences," she says. "I did this for many months until the magazine was in shreds. When I started school, I used the *National Geographic* magazines in the library to the same effect. It was the only place you could see pictures of naked bodies."

Daryl went to boarding school in the seventh grade and had roommates who all masturbated. "After lights out, you could hear those sheets popping," she recalls. "I was enormously relieved to know that many other girls my age masturbated, too. I had gotten the message that it was a no-no, but just couldn't believe that something that felt so good could be bad."

Pauline relates her childhood masturbation experiences:

I remember at age nine repeating the word "mas-tur-ba-tion" with my sisters in the back of our station wagon so that I could learn to pronounce this big new word. Yet, I was totally oblivious to the real meaning until I got to college. I thought that getting off under the faucet in the bathtub was my own little game, and that stroking my skin gently with my fingers (which equally turned me on) was actually the taboo my big sisters told me "masturbation" was. Despite my lack of understanding of the definition of masturbation, I practiced it at every opportunity.

The common thread here is that most young children discover masturbation on their own, that it feels so good and so right, but for some mysterious reason, it is considered bad or dangerous and is strictly forbidden.

A BRIEF HISTORY OF MASTURBATION

Of all of the sexual activities that people engage in, masturbation has consistently been the most frequently employed, secret, and maligned. Physicians and philosophers in ancient China believed that ejaculation from masturbation was a waste of vital *chi,* or energy, and the first sexuality advice manuals written by Taoist masters condemned men from doing it. Early Taoists understood that women ejaculated, too (see page 117), but female emissions weren't thought to be as vital as men's, so female masturbation wasn't specifically prohibited. Early Indian Tantric gurus also believed that sperm took forty days to produce (it takes sixty-three days) and should therefore not be wasted.[83]

Autoeroticism, as masturbation was referred to in classical Greece, was considered to be a favorite pastime of the mythical satyrs who embodied the baser side of human nature. While masturbation was not prohibited for humans, that is, men, it was derided as an activity more appropriate to slaves than masters who had "real" sex with boys and prostitutes.[84]

Hysteria, a complex of symptoms that includes fainting, edema (fluid or blood trapped in the genitals—the female version of "blue balls"), nervousness, irritability, weight loss, and depression, was reported in Egypt as early as 2000 B.C.E. and was apparently prevalent in Greece as well. Greek physicians often performed genital massage on their patients with the (accurate) belief that orgasm would bring some temporary relief.[85] One might term this practice "professional masturbation." In desperation, some women surely masturbated themselves, or a close female friend may have lent a hand, but we'll never know the extent of this solitary masturbatory practice.

The early Christians roundly condemned homosexuality, which they saw as going hand-in-hand (as it were) with mutual and solitary masturbation. Nuns who were caught using dildos were treated especially harshly. By the Middle Ages, Catholic authorities aggressively prohibited masturbation and any other sexual activity that was not performed in the service of marital fidelity, meaning reproduction. Medieval physicians were particularly concerned about masturbation by monks and virgins, and recommended a host of debilitating remedies including bleeding, ascetic diets or fasting, flagellation, cold baths, sitting on stones, and the deliberate suppression of fantasies.[86]

The Old Testament, however, does not forbid masturbation, as is commonly believed. In chapter 38 of Genesis, Onan was required by Jewish custom to marry his brother's widow to provide a child to inherit the family property. *The New Annotated Bible* passage reads, "since Onan knew that the offspring would not be his, he spilled his semen on the ground whenever he went in to his brother's wife so that he would not give offspring to his brother."[87] Onan, one of the most widely reviled biblical characters, was put to death, not because he masturbated alone, but because he apparently practiced withdrawal instead of fathering children that would not legally be his. It was only in the eighteenth century that the story of Onan was reinterpreted by theologians to prohibit masturbation, or "onanism," as it came to be known. In 1710, the anonymously published book *On the Heinous Sin of Self-Pollution, and All Its Frightful Consequences, in both Sexes, Consider'd with Spiritual and Physical Advice to Those, who have already injur'd themselves by this abominable practice. And seasonable Admonition to the Youth of the Nation, (of both Sexes) and those whose Tuition they are under, whether Parents, Guardians, Masters, or Mistresses* launched the modern campaign against masturbation. The title says it all. Another classic antimasturbation tract of the period is *Onanism: A Treatise on the Diseases Produced by Masturbation, Or, the Dangerous Effects of Secret and Excessive Venery,* by the Swiss physician Simon A. A. D. Tissot, who proclaimed that the loss of "vital fluid" through masturbation could cause mental illness, among a host of other bodily ills.[88] According to historian Sara Matthews Grieco, the eighteenth century was an era in which "doctors, pedagogues, and parents participated in a collective delirium of repression" against masturbation "that would reach its peak in the 19th century."[89] The Victorians took up the crusade against "self-abuse" and the "pollution of moral purity" with unparalleled vigor. Even feminists like Mary Wollstonecraft warned against "the nasty habits of schoolgirls," which she feared would be carried into later life, where they might unduly influence the prescribed asexuality of proper Victorian women.[90]

Two of America's most widely known food products produced in the 19th century—Graham Crackers and Kellogg's Cornflakes—were aggressively promoted by their crusading developers as "pure" foods that would not promote untoward tendencies in children. Sylvester Graham, a minister who preached vegetarianism and athleticism along with Christianity, warned against the loss of "vital fluids" from masturbation, advocating foods made from whole wheat "Graham" flour in place of meat and spicy foods. He also promoted sleeping on wooden beds to suppress masturbatory urges in boys.[91] Cornflake magnate J. H. Kellogg listed thirty-nine signs that a boy was masturbating, including poor posture, acne, bashfulness, nail-biting, and bed-wetting. For recidivists, he recommended draconian measures that included suturing the foreskin over the glans to prevent erection for boys, and pouring "pure carbolic acid to the clitoris," for girls. Parents went to great lengths to prevent their children from "polluting" themselves, following Kellogg's advice to bandage their genitals or hands.[92] These strategies against childhood masturbation were still widely prevalent in the twentieth century. Mary Steichen Calderone, a physician and cofounder of the Sexuality Information and Education Council of the United States (SIECUS), often said that when she was a child in the 1920s, her parents forced her to wear aluminum mittens to bed to prevent her from masturbating.

In spite of these efforts, masturbation remained a popular if secret activity. Alfred Kinsey's studies during the late 1940s and early 1950s found that 94 percent of men and 40 percent of women had masturbated to orgasm.[93] *Sex in America*, a broad-based national survey published in 1994, reports that 60 percent of adult men and 40 percent of adult women say that they masturbated in the past year; 25 percent of men and 10 percent of women say that they do so at least once a week. This survey also found that women and men who engage in frequent partner sex are also the ones who masturbate the most regularly.

Betty Dodson, an artist and sexuality educator, was the first person to promote the use of vibrators to enhance masturbation. In

1971, Dodson began holding sexuality consciousness-raising sessions and self-published the booklet *Liberating Masturbation,* later updated, expanded, and reissued as *Sex for One.*[94] Soon Dodson began holding her famous Bodysex workshops in which she exuberantly promoted genital pride and masturbation as a primary form of sexual expression, rather than as a crutch until the next partner comes along.

Lonnie Barbach and other West Coast sex educators began advocating masturbation to help women learn to have orgasms. Barbach published *For Yourself: The Fulfillment of Female Sexuality.*[95] Like *Sex for One*, the book became a classic and has remained in print since. Shere Hite asked about masturbation in the questionnaire that she distributed to over 100,000 women in the early 1970s, and in her best-selling *Hite Report,* women poured out their feelings on the subject for over 150 pages.[96] These books were all internationally distributed and became critical in beginning to rescue masturbation from silence and shame.

In the 1970s and 1980s, for the first time in human history, self-pleasuring was openly acknowledged as a significant and healthy sexual activity. As women's sexual autonomy increased through contraception, abortion, divorce, and economic independence during the 1990s, though, masturbation once again came under attack due to pressure from the religious right in Congress and fundamentalist advocacy groups. President Bill Clinton fired his Surgeon General Joycelyn Elders for agreeing (not for *advocating*, as the media repeatedly misreported) that information on masturbation should be included in teenage sex education courses. Masturbation is rarely mentioned as a significant means of self-pleasuring or a self-discovery technique in the new government-funded "abstinence only" sexuality education programs across the country. (See page 28).

Psychologist Leonore Tiefer believes that "masturbation symbolizes all the primary problems that the Christian Right has with sexuality: it represents sex for pleasure rather than procreation, and because it's done in secret by children and adults, it's not subject to external control." She adds, "they believe that the Bible prohibits it." Tiefer suspects that the real focus of this attack is on girls, because anything that enhances women's autonomy threatens the male order. "I think we can estimate the success or failure of the right's influence on sexuality by how masturbation seems to be going. Right now, it's going badly."[97]

In response to this dismal state of affairs, Good Vibrations, Grand Opening!, and Toys in Babeland, three well-known women-friendly sex boutiques, instituted the First National Masturbate-A-Thon on May 7, 1999. They solicit pledges as for a walkathon, but for minutes of masturbation. The proceeds are divided among several organizations that promote AIDS awareness and services.

MASTURBATION FOREVER!

Masturbation is defined as any kind of sexual stimulation that does not include coitus. This means touching oneself on the breasts, genitals, or any other part of the body in a way that is intended to elicit sexual feelings or sensations. To keep masturbation interesting, people not only use hands, vibrators, dildos, or other sex toys, but add an astounding variety of objects including feathers, rubber gloves, whipped cream and other foodstuffs, cat-o-nine-tails, even whips and other instruments and apparatus traditionally used in S/M games. There is also mutual masturbation, in which a couple stimulates each other with or without having intercourse. What does this mean for lesbians who have very real and sexually rewarding experiences? Or for gay men, or even for heterosexual couples who do everything but put a penis in the vagina or anus? Aren't they having sex? Perhaps there is no such thing as masturbation—just sex with or without intercourse. (See Greta Christina's ruminations on this subject on page 132.)

Numerous studies have shown that for many women, masturbation results in orgasm more reliably than does intercourse, and typically it produces stronger orgasms to boot. Masturbation has countless benefits. It helps you to discover the types of stimulation you like best. You're in complete control of the amount and type of stimulation that you prefer. You don't need contraception or STD protection. It is sex when you want it, and it can provide stress reduction, menstrual cramp relief, and even a cardiovascular workout if you do it for a long enough period of time and have many orgasms. Sexual activity produces the body's natural opiate, endorphins, as well as hormones that can enhance mood and increase a sense of well-being. Some people masturbate to increase their desire for sex. As Truman Capote once said, "You don't have to dress up for it."[98] In an after-dinner speech delivered to the Parisian "Stomach Club" in 1879, Mark Twain cited a reference to masturbation from Julius Caesar's *Commentaries:* "To the lonely it is company; to the forsaken it is a friend; to the aged and impotent it is a benefactor; they that be penniless are yet rich, in that they still have this majestic diversion."[99]

HOW WE DO IT

There is no right or wrong way to masturbate, but the variations seem quite endless. Wanda found vibrators too harsh, so she adapted an electric toothbrush quite handily. Some women masturbate as frequently as once or more a day to achieve what Jill calls "maintenance orgasms." In a survey done for *The Good Vibrations Guide to Sex,* Cathy Winks and Anne Semans found that people tend to change their masturbation habits when they are with a partner.[100] Some people felt that they didn't need to masturbate with a partner, while others didn't want their partners to know that they masturbate. It seems that while many women may have recovered from the guilt of solitary masturbation, many are still too uncomfortable or feel too guilty to share this sex-enhancing activity with a partner.

There are women who get a particular thrill from secretly masturbating in public places. LuAnn says that she often does it on the train during her long, boring commute to work, strategically placing a coat or sweater across her lap. "If no one is sitting beside me," she explains. Edna and her boyfriend like to masturbate each other at rock concerts with hands in each other's pockets. They both suspect that they aren't the only ones. Rachael, a magazine editor, recalls one particularly memorable orgasm of the "look-ma-no-hands" variety in the fifth row at Carnegie Hall to Beethoven's Ninth.

Despite unrelenting efforts to erase masturbation throughout history, it shows us time and again that it is ubiquitous. According to *The Complete Dictionary of Sexology*, some 95 percent of men and 85 percent of women masturbate, at least occasionally.[101]

VIVA LA VIBRATOR

In *The Technology of Orgasm: "Hysteria," the Vibrator, and Women's Sexual Satisfaction*, Rachel Maines documents the secret history of the vibrator, and revealed that once electric models were available around 1880, they were widely advertised in needlework magazines, appliance catalogs, and Sears and Roebuck catalogs, marketed as a sexual health aid.[102] The mass marketing of vibrators relieved physicians and midwives from having to treat women suffering from "hysteria," or sexual depravation, with labor-intensive genital massage. Sometime after 1930, advertisements for vibrators disappeared. Maines surmises that this may have been attributable to their frequent appearance in pornographic films.

The vibrator resurfaced in the 1960s, and this time, Maines notes, "few efforts were made to camouflage its sexual benefits." Nonetheless, she shows that many sex therapists, and even feminists, were slow to endorse the sexual independence that vibrators gave women.

More than anyone else, Betty Dodson is responsible for reclaiming the humble vibrator from the electronic dustbin. Dodson says that many women still hold the romantic fantasy of Prince Charming leaning over and kissing them awake, and the two of them living happily after. "In my version, Sleeping Beauty wakes herself up with a 60-hertz electric massager vibrating at 5,000 revolutions per minute," she says. "This activity can be shared with a lover, unless he or she has fallen asleep after they've had their orgasm."[103]

In contrast to the widespread use of vibrators in the late nineteenth and early twentieth centuries, laws controlling sex toys—especially vibrators—were enacted in the 1950s, greatly impeding their distribution. Many models continued to be sold in drug and department stores, but only as "massagers."

Vibrators now come in an astonishing variety of shapes and colors, including penis-shaped, ribbed, or "smoothies," straight, bent, egg-shaped, animal-shaped, or balls. Some can be quite fanciful with faces that have lips or tongues molded on the tips, and appended to serve as extra stimulation to the clitoral glans while the body is inside of the vagina, in direct contact with other clitoral structures. There are battery-powered and plug-in models each with its advantages and disadvantages. Battery-powered models are noisier but tend to be cheaper and smaller, and you can use them on a camping trip or in countries that have an incompatible electrical voltage. Some battery vibrators are waterproof, designed for bathing, or cavorting in a hot tub or cool mountain stream. There are battery-run strap-ons for those who want or need hands-free vibration, and smaller ones for anal stimulation.

Electric vibrators are larger, quieter, more powerful, and there are no batteries to run down mid-climax, but you can't use them everywhere. Most electric models have two speeds, medium and high, but some have a slide or dial mechanism that allows you to vary the speed from a low purr to a hearty roar. Vibrator aficionados often have impressive collections on hand for any occasion. Good Vibrations, which began as a vibrator store, reports that the battery-operated Crystal Jelly G Spot Vibe is their number-one seller.

If you're not sure about which type of vibrator to buy, or aren't satisfied with your current model, check out Joani Blank's *Good Vibrations: The Complete Guide to Vibrators*.[104] In addition to detailed information on how to choose, use, and maintain your vibrator, Blank offers a number of suggestions on how to integrate the use of a vibrator with a partner.

My friend Susan explains how she and her husband use a vibrator routinely:

> I learned the pleasures of a vibrator when I was without a partner and for a long time thought it was just for pleasuring myself and at first I was a bit hesitant to tell my partner, now my husband, about my high-speed friend. Luckily he and I were able to talk about what felt good and what our fantasies were. I told him that using the vibrator was like having another lover in the bed with us... a turn on for both of us. I especially like to use the vibrator on my clitoris while he fucks me. We also like to use it for massage, it feels great on sore necks and shoulders and can get you in the mood when you use it on the buttocks and inner thigh.

As long as we look at sex as a performance, many partners may continue to feel threatened or inadequate when a woman wants to introduce a vibrator as an extra hand, as it were, into lovemaking. If the goal is pleasure rather than performance, than the threat is removed, and sex becomes a journey of discovery rather than revelation. Susan took a smart approach and talked about it with her husband. Not surprisingly, they found common ground.

TOYS FOR GIRLS

The word "dildo" means "artificial penis," and as such, dildos have been in use for at least 6,000 years and probably much longer. In addition to phallic-shaped objects, realistically carved dildos fashioned from leather, wood, bone, or stone have been found at archaeological sites dating as far back as 4000 B.C.E. A number of well-preserved examples have been recovered, including one from the Varna site in present-day Bulgaria, with a tip of hammered gold, and an exquisitely carved double "phallic baton" found in France that bears a striking resemblance to modern-day sex toys intended for use by two women.[105]

Today, dildos are made from silicon, rubber, vinyl, or lucite for both vaginal and anal insertion, and there appears to be one designed to suit every requirement, taste, whimsy, fantasy, and predilection. Some dildos are amazingly lifelike, exhibiting molded glans, bulging veins, and scrotum, and tend to come in large to extra large. Millions are sold every year.

Dildos also come in many colors, from pinkish, lavender, brown, jet-black, and rainbow, to colorful translucent jellies with bubbles, to crystal clear. While manufacturers eventually responded to consumer demand for multihued skin tones, providing café au lait, chocolate, and black, salespeople in sex boutiques report that many people actually prefer colors that contrast with their own skin color. Dildos may be straight, curved, bent, double-tipped, rippled, ribbed, or smooth. Apparently there is no accounting for what will appeal to customers. Some women prefer the demure smoothies, while others unabashedly like the veiny bumps-and-all versions—and the bigger, the better.

The very definition of dildo implies an *erect* penis, but the newest wrinkle in faux penises is Mr. Softie, a squishy, pale-pink rendition of a flaccid penis that looks incredibly lifelike, feels marvelously pliable, and stretches several feet only to snap back to its limp state. "I'd like one as a teaching tool," says Isa, who teaches health at a New York City high school, "because men don't walk around with this ramrod straight, ten-inch erection in real life. This would be much more realistic."

Some states such as Texas still have laws prohibiting the sale of devices intended for genital stimulation. The state has a law against the sale of sex toys, which was only recently modified to allow their purchase for "medical reasons."

"Will residents need a note from their doctors to buy a dildo?" Cathy Winks and Anne Semans muse. "Where are they supposed to buy dildos—from a pharmacy or an adult book store?" In the spring of 1999, conservative Alabama legislators passed a law forbidding the sale of "any obscene material or any device designed or marketed as useful primarily for the stimulation of human genital organs." The maximum penalty for flouting this law: a year in jail and a $10,000 fine. Predictably, this law was challenged in court and ultimately deemed unconstitutional. Had it remained in force, cows in Alabama would have had more rights to use vibrators (apparently employed by farmers as an artificial insemination aid) than women. The debate made national news, and was the butt of numerous late-night talk show jokes. While laughable and nonsensical, this bald attempt by Christian fundamentalists to impose regressive standards on sexuality is yet another skirmish in the ongoing sex wars and should not be taken lightly. If we value our sexual freedom, we should work to overturn these antiquated laws because, in the end, they are aimed at controlling women, especially lesbians, as well as gay men who do not conform to the male heterosexual model of sexuality.

In spite of the ready availability of sex toys, many women still feel tentative or guilty about buying and using them. The fear of anyone finding an eight-inch lavender penis in the sock drawer, be it your lover or mother, still inspires anxiety in many of us, and grabs our hand as we write down our credit card number on an order form.

On Our Backs, the famous clits-up lesbian sexzine, asked women, "What's the most embarrassing experience involving your sex toy?" and learned:

Natalie... put her dildo in the microwave. Forty-one percent of women had a dildo break during use.... a bag of dildos got searched at the airport.... a straight friend found a dildo under the bed.... parents came in while a dildo was sitting on the kitchen table.... a finger got stuck in a vibrator while trying to fix the battery... got pussy burns from falling asleep with the vibrator on... and... one woman's vibrator turned on in her backpack at the bus stop!

Most sex toys are designed by men (like so many other items we use), so the magazine asked women how they would design a fantasy toy. They answered:

A dildo that satisfies both partners.... better straps for harness so there's no slipping.... a toy that sucks.... a toy that licks all around.... an anal and cunt dildo.... a dildo with as much control as hands... and... a long-handled dildo for women with short arms.[106]

In addition to vibrators and dildos, there is an endless range of sex toys readily available through sexuality boutiques and catalogs. Women-friendly shops and catalogs are listed in Resources beginning on page 235.

FANTASIES AND ROLE PLAYING

People have probably always employed private or shared fantasies to make sex more exciting. Fantasies make the forbidden, the foolish, the wild and wooly accessible, and in situations where sex is impossible, forbidden, an obligation, or lackluster, fantasies often save the day. For many people, fantasies fill an otherwise hopeless void, and if their imagination is rich and free enough, they can be as orgasmic alone as they can with a partner, sometimes more reliably and powerfully so. Before women began redefining sex for themselves, fantasies were a subversive way of rewriting male scripts. In secret scenarios, women were not only the actors, but the casting consultants, the costume designers, architects of the set, and directors. Then as now, we can have sex with whomever we please, anywhere we want, and ask our beloved to do anything we want just exactly the way we like it. We can do things in our waking dreams, like have sex on the wing of an airplane, in shark-infested waters, or on a bench at the mall. If only real life could be like this. Well, sometimes it actually can.

Fantasies can be funny, somber, daring, scary, wicked, or raunchy, and may provide a few minutes of escape from the mundane; they may promote heightened pleasure or be truly revelatory. "My World of the Unknown," a short story by Egyptian writer Alifa Rifaat, is one of the most poignant examples of how powerful and transformative fantasies can be, especially for women in sexually repressive cultures.[107] The husband of the nameless narrator is transferred to a site far removed from the beloved familiarity of Cairo. On her first house-hunting venture, she is taken by an abandoned house that is said to be haunted by *djinn,* a celestial spirit, which may appear in animal or spirit form. She feels strangely drawn to the empty house and overgrown garden, and against the advice of the realtor, she rents it. After the family settles in, she withdraws from social life and focuses on her garden where one day she observes an exotic multicolored snake in a tree. "I felt a current of radiation from its eyes that penetrated to my heart," explains the narrator. She continues:

> I rose from my place, overwhelmed by the feeling that I was on the brink of a new world, a new destiny, or rather, if you wish, the threshold of a new love.... I began to be intoxicated by the soft musical whisperings. I felt her cool and soft and smooth, her coldness producing a painful convulsion in my body and hurting me to the point of terror. I felt her as she slipped between the covers, then her two tiny fangs, like two pearls, began to caress my body; arriving at my thighs, the golden tongue, like an arak twig, inserted its pronged tip between them and began sipping and exhaling, sipping the poisons of my desire and exhaling the nectar of my ecstasy, 'til

my whole body tingled and started to shake in sharp, painful, rapturous spasms—and all the while the tenderest of words were whispered to me as I confided to her all my longings.[108]

Through this vivid and powerfully moving fantasy, the narrator is able to transcend the constraints of her phallocentric culture and realize in a meaningful way her right to sexual pleasure.

Nancy Friday's collections of other women's sexual fantasies (see Resources) give us a clear idea of their breadth and depth, dispelling the myth that men's fantasies are more active and powerful. In the introduction to her third book, *Women on Top,* Friday observes a striking change in women's fantasies from those in her earlier volumes. "More than any other emotion, guilt determined the story lines of the fantasies in *My Secret Garden*." In order to get past it, women fantasized about rape, bodily harm, humiliation, and, most frequently, had fantasy sex with faceless strangers. This worked, Friday suggests, to preserve the "nice girl" image in women's own minds. But in *Women on Top,* she found "women's voices finally dealing with the full lexicon of human emotion, sexual imagery, and language."[109]

The male-centered, intercourse-focused model of sexuality has begun to change, and this is happening only because women are asserting their right to equal pleasure during sex. For many women and their partners, de-emphasizing intercourse is the first step in the journey to deeper, more rewarding, even transformative sexual experiences. Claiming masturbation as a legitimate part of our birthright—for self-pleasure and as well as an essential means of sexual discovery—is the next step. Using sex toys, fantasies, games, and visual and written erotica can help us in our sexual exploration. For women who want more, there are workshops such as the ones described in chapter 5 that can help us learn about our anatomy; work through our inhibitions; act out our fantasies in a safe environment; try new techniques; share our fears, breakthroughs, and triumphs firsthand with others; and receive in return advice, support, and encouragement.

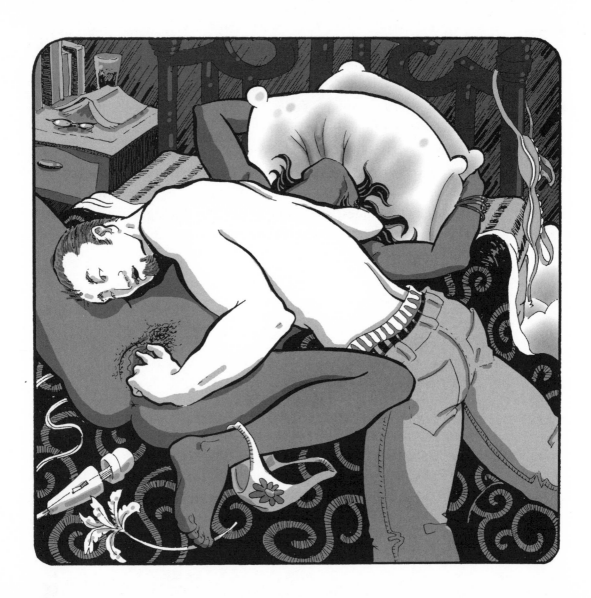

BEYOND INTERCOURSE
New Erotic Possibilities

5

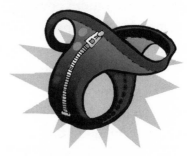

Now, at the dawn of the twenty-first century, the male-centered heterosexual model of sexuality described at the beginning of chapter 1 is undergoing a dramatic transformation.

While intercourse has previously been the centerpiece of sex per the male-centered heterosexual model, the very definition of sex is changing in our favor, encompassing pretty much anything that we feel is sexual. Indeed, many people now acknowledge that sex encompasses far more than vaginal intercourse, although the definition of what sex is will probably always remain somewhat fluid.

What if intercourse were no longer the centerpiece of sexual activity? What would it be like? Would sex seem more like work instead of play? Certainly not, if you are willing to think about sex in a different way. Would men get bored during sex? Probably not, as we will soon see. Would men still get *their* orgasms? Of course, and they may be even more powerful and exuberant than ever before. Would relationships fall apart? No way! Increasing sexual options can only heighten sexual response, enliven lackluster sex, enhance desire, deepen intimacy, and strengthen sexual bonds between partners.

This is not to say that intercourse should not still be a pleasurable sexual activity, but instead that it be de-emphasized in favor of a variety of techniques that are more rewarding for women. Men and women need to engage in a more lengthy erotic give-and-take that postpones orgasm and results in ever escalating levels of sexual excitement. This includes incorporating masturbation, vibrators, sex toys, fantasies, and videos or written erotica, as well as kissing, cuddling, caressing, holding hands, dancing, hot talk, role playing, and safe, consensual S/M games. Even verbal stimulation, which may or may not lead to orgasm, can be both sexual and sexually satisfying.

Many women and men are already making this leap by taking classes, workshops, or going through experiential training to actualize their unexplored fantasies and expand the range of how they perceive what is sexy and stimulating. Such sessions may include information on anatomy and physiology, exercises to enhance body awareness, demonstrations of Tantric and Taoist sexual practices, hands-on instruction in erotic massage and masturbatory techniques, dressing up, talking hot, and role playing.

ADAPTING ANCIENT SEXUAL RITES FOR THE NEW MILLENNIUM

The intercourse-centered model of sex is so deeply rooted in our culture that we find it difficult to imagine a time when it was not the norm. Yet we have to look no further than the modern sexual practices of our oldest spiritual belief systems, Chinese Taoism and the Indian Tantric tradition, to find a non-intercourse model right on our doorstep.

The first sexuality advice books by Taoists were written about 600 B.C.E., and by Tantric sages in India about 300 C.E. They were based upon the oral traditions of earlier pagan cultures in which women were revered, even worshiped for their miraculous ability to conceive and give birth. This life-giving phenomenon was directly associated with their sexuality, and sexuality, in turn, was probably the central sacrament of life, the thread that connected birth to life, death and rebirth, and was believed to be the holy rite that inferred "enlightenment," the bridge between the human and the divine. Anthropological evidence suggests that elaborate sexual rituals were acted out in temples illuminated by fire and perfumed by incense. The participants probably wore special clothing and jewelry, meditated, engaged in visualization, and practiced breathing techniques designed to promote the circulation of sexual energy throughout the entire body. They feasted, drank beer and wine, ingested hallucinogens, and performed ecstatic dancing accompanied by chanting, singing, or drumming. In this ancient model, women's sexual pleasure was considered paramount, a sacred responsibility to be enthusiastically fulfilled, and in the process, both or all participants reached an altered state of consciousness, which could have been interpreted as "enlightenment."

It's surprising how closely modern sexual practices mimic these ancient ceremonies. Instead of leopard-skin robes, we might wear little black cocktail dresses or sequined gowns, sexy lingerie, or trendy tank tops and jeans. Instead of necklaces of bear claws or tigers' teeth, we might wear diamonds, pearls, or birthstones, or even lapis lazuli, the favored gem of ancient priestesses, or cowrie shells, which in prehistoric times were seen as potent symbols of the holy vulva. We might wine and dine our sweetie, dance our brains out in clubs lit by flashing lights, or we might perform erotic dances for each other in the privacy of our bedrooms perfumed with incense and lit by candles or a fireplace. Instead of chanting or singing, we might turn on our favorite music, and in place of visualization, we might share our sexual fantasies and exchange erotic massages. The romantics among us might even read a bit of poetry. In place of public sex, which in the distant past would have served as a powerful aphrodisiac, we might watch a sexy video to rekindle or enhance desire, or videotape ourselves making love. When we do any of these things, we are reenacting sexual rituals as old as time itself.

Today, there are people who practice strict "orthodox" Tantra or Taoist rituals that provide spiritual sustenance as well as sexual pleasures, while others adapt the sexual elements more freely to explore their sexual potential and discover the rewards of full-body sexual response. During sex, partners may dress up (or down) for each other, do rhythmic breathing together, and gaze deeply into each other's eyes. They may feed each other and have some wine or other ceremonial drink. Then they may share intimate secrets, thoughts, and fantasies. Every part of the body, from the earlobes to the toes, is caressed or massaged. Orthodox Tantric and Taoist practices utilize dozens of specific positions, but in the modern generic forms, variety and inventiveness are encouraged. Stimulation is varied, intensified, and withdrawn so that both partners progressively reach higher levels of sexual arousal while the man consciously avoids ejaculation. Only when the woman has had as much pleasure and as many orgasms as she wants is the man brought to orgasm with or without penetration. Thus, sex, which is normally initiated and concluded within five to fifteen minutes, may last anywhere from thirty to forty minutes to two or three hours. The idea is that both partners will reach the point of satiation, beyond which they cannot go further. This satiation certainly won't happen every time.

Not to worry: Quickies still have their place. But given that sex has a special place in modern relationships, and is perceived by many as a healthy and emotionally rewarding recreational activity, why not put forth the effort to make it more worthwhile?

LEARNING EJACULATORY CONTROL

By the time men are out of their teens, many are psychologically and physically conditioned to go for orgasm, and some may initially have trouble modifying this pattern. At first, some men may even experience the loss of erection as they pass their usual time frame for ejaculation, and this may cause feelings of panic and an unwillingness to learn to postpone it. In this case, it might be useful to practice alone, perhaps for a few months, before trying this technique with a partner. For men who find new patterns too difficult to master alone, there are teachers of Tantra or Tao all over the country who can provide expert help, one-on-one, or through workshops (see Resources). The Body Electric School (see my account on page 186) also has a wide range of workshops designed to help men learn ejaculatory control and explore full-body sexual response.

A man's ability to control and postpone ejaculation is the key to longer and more satisfying sex. There are a number of strategies that men can use to accomplish this and they all hark directly back to early Taoist and Tantric sexual techniques. To avoid going too far too quickly, it's essential to vary the type and amount of stimulation of the penis. If you are using hands, lighten up and use the tongue, or rub the penis against the thigh for less intense stimulation. Fantasize for a bit. Measured breathing can also help control the heart rate, which rises as ejaculation approaches, and contracting the pelvic floor muscles (the ones that can stop the flow of urine) may temporarily disrupt the intensity of nerve signals that lead to ejaculation. Squeezing the penis at its base or pressing firmly on the perineum and pulling the testicles down and away from the body are other techniques that can interrupt or modulate the escalation of nerve impulses. During intercourse, men should try to stop thrusting until the urge to ejaculate passes. There is no right or wrong way to postpone ejaculation. It is critical that men avoid the approach of the "moment of ejaculatory inevitability," when he can no longer avoid orgasm.

Most experts agree that spectacular sex isn't something that just happens, but rather is consciously cultivated. Under the male-centered, heterosexual model of sexuality, men feel a sense of failure if they can't "get it up," "get it in," and "get it off." But according to the Tantric and Taoist models, men are considered failures when they don't put their partner's pleasure first and provide the types of stimulation that lead to her sexual satisfaction. Early sexuality manuals offer detailed advice on how a man can tell if he is pleasing his partner: she lifts her body, she is panting, her perspiration is copious, her face flushes, her voice is shaking, she can't speak, her expression looks bewitched, or as the Taoist master Wu Hsien notes, "the pulses of her vulva become noticeable and her secretions are flooding." These are signs of a woman in the throes of full-blown sexual response, a state that is not easily achieved for many women under the intercourse model. Wu presciently observed that women are "slow to be aroused/But also slow to be satiated."

DISCOVERING NEW EROTIC POSSIBILITIES

Betty Dodson's Bodysex seminars evolved from a series of consciousness-raising groups focused on women's sexuality that she facilitated in the early 1970s. In the earliest groups, women shared their frustrations, uncertainties, and questions about sexuality. After a while, Dodson decided to teach "masturbation by demonstration" to allow women to see a real female orgasm. The demonstration was so successful that it became a regular feature of the workshops. In these sessions, women undressed; explored and admired their bodies and genitals; learned masturbatory techniques, anal massage, and erotic massage; and ultimately performed the female version of the "circle jerk," reveling in self-discovery and liberation from the secrecy and taboos surrounding female sexuality. The Bodysex groups became legendary and provided the model for the modern experiential workshop. In 1990, after doing Bodysex workshops across the country for twenty years, Dodson made a breakthrough video of a workshop to more widely distribute the information and experience of participating in a session (see Resources). Today she does private sex coaching, occasional advanced workshops for sex therapists and manages her informative Web site (see Resources).

INDIVIDUAL SEX COACHING

Sue, a manager in a large global corporation and twice divorced, is fifty-three years old. She decided that she would like to have an outstanding sex life without a partner so that she could have more satisfying sex with a partner when the opportunity arrives. Sue took an individual two-hour coaching session from Dodson, and found the experience to be transformative:

> Until now, I had only masturbated by tensing up my whole body, holding my breath, and holding my arm across my stomach (which I now know blocked the flow of sexual energy that moves up and through the entire body). I used this same posture when my lovers would manually bring me to orgasm. It was very helpful to have Betty imitate the "stiff posture" I had used for orgasm for forty years. She showed me how I would look if I were dancing with that posture. Egads! It was

THE ROOTS OF TAO AND TANTRA

Taoism grew out of prehistoric pagan cultures in China whose worldview focused on the interconnectedness of humans and the natural world, and the mystical relationships between them. "Tao" means "the way," and the basic assumption underlying this belief system is that body and soul are infused with "chi," or energy, which moves one along the path toward harmony with nature and ultimately, immortality. According to the Tao, "chi" consists of "yin," female attributes, complemented by "yang," the male essence. Both elements are present in women and men. Sex is a sacred rite that permits the union of yin and yang, and prolonged ecstatic sexual activity circulates chi to the higher centers of the heart and the brain, enabling mortals to find the way to the divine.

The roots of Tantra, the ancient Eastern Indian spiritual tradition, can be traced to goddess-worshiping cults in the Sumer region. Their beliefs centered on the celebration of the ebb and flow of the seasons, reincarnation, the veneration of animals, and the powerful but occult interconnections between the natural world and the cosmos. Sexuality was seen as the means to access these mystical connections and unravel the enigmas of the universe. Yoga, especially kundalini (female energy), was originally highly sexual in nature and its complex rituals were designed to enable humans to transcend earthly existence and become one with the divine.

While Tantra flourished in India, goddess worship was gradually replaced by authoritarian male deities in Greek, Hebraic, and Islamic cultures. Earlier cults venerated women and viewed sexuality as a sacred ritual that revealed the divine in each person, but the new patriarchal mythologies drew a sharp and unbreachable distinction between the body and the spirit. At the heart of this dualistic philosophy is the concept that we are born as a result of sex, which is innately sinful, and consequently must spend our lives striving for forgiveness for this "original sin." Sex is perceived to be a dangerous part of our humanity that marks us with a blot that can only be erased or forgiven after death. This deeply colors how we look at sexuality today.

Interest in Tantra and Taoism has waxed and waned in Western culture since the Middle Ages, and various elements have been interpreted and adapted by many practitioners over time. Radical therapists and philosophers fled Europe during World War II, and many settled in California, where they employed various aspects of these belief systems in the foundation of the human potential movement in the United States. The Beat generation of the 1950s delved into Eastern mysticism and challenged the rigid social and sexual standards of the day, helping to pave the way for the sexual revolution of the 1960s.

Nik Douglas, a leading scholar of Tantra, recalls the fascination with Asian mysticism in the sixties. "Tantric symbols appeared everywhere, on T-shirts, buttons, posters, and on record albums. Mandalas appeared on pop concert posters. Tantric art designs were painted on several of the Beatles' cars. Jimi Hendrix had Tantric Yantra diagrams painted on his guitar and on his cheeks." Yet Douglas notes that the 1960s' version of Tantric sexuality was essentially male-focused, promising "enhanced sexual potency for men, of hour-long orgasms or ecstasies for him." Douglas asserts that it was not until the flowering of the New Age movement in the 1980s that "women started to take up the challenge that Tantra teachings so radically promoted: the role of woman as the embodiment of the Great Goddess, sexually liberated and multiorgasmic."

helpful to see a visual representation of how I have suppressed my sexual energy all these years.

Betty recommended setting up an inviting environment, using candles, which produce a delicious soft touch and music which promotes fantasies and encourages movement. I had always used "mood" music, but I guess I've been in a rut all these years in that respect also. She also suggested keeping the musical beat varied and including some more intense rhythms to enhance mood and movement during the session and I was surprised at the great music that she provided.

Betty also encouraged the use of fantasies, which promote both the desire for sex and the intensity of the experience. One I have had is about fucking wild beasts, which may come from a childhood memory of watching dogs fuck. Another recalls when a high school boyfriend is penetrating just slightly, not really inside. In my fantasies, I could be the man (my masculine side of my personality, which all women have) or I could be the woman "desired" by a man. I've been into some S&M and found it a turn-on, so Betty recommended works by A. N. Roquelaure (a pen name of vampire doyenne Anne Rice) and her *Beauty* series. She also suggested renting pornography/

erotica videos and scanning through the "story" to get to the stimulating parts. She said that many women prefer videos made for gay men, because you don't have to sit through a "story" to get to the sexy parts. They go for the gold!

The heart of Betty's session is genital massage. She uses massage oil rather than lube because it isn't as messy, is good for your skin, and has a sexy odor. I chose Charlie Sunshine's secret formula because I love the tantalizing smell of vanilla. We started by examining my genitals and I looked at them *for the first time in my life*. Betty said that my vulva had a diamond shape and helped me appreciate the uniqueness of the visible parts. Then she showed me different types of strokes to do with my hands. One is a kind of scissor stroke in which you press the glans, shaft, and inner lips of the clitoris between two fingers pulling up and down. With the other hand, you can knead the lower abdomen just above the pubic hairline.

Essentially, you have three "events" going at once to build up muscle tension in the genitals and the rest of the body. Before you begin to masturbate, you do ten or more contractions of the PC muscles, tensing only the genital area, not the abdomen or the buttocks. Then you take some long, slow breaths, sucking your breath in like you are sipping hot tea and making "ah…ha…" sounds as you exhale.

Then you add the "pelvic rock," sort of rolling the pelvis backward and forth without lifting your butt off the floor. You can also try making circles with your pelvis, or any other motion that feels good. When you are very excited you can try lifting the entire lower back off the floor, which creates tension in the thigh area, but this is too hard to sustain for the whole session. Betty changed the type/tempo of the music to go with different "beats." The idea is to loosen up and have fun using varied types of stimulation to keep sexual tension from exploding too fast. Combining all three movements, PC muscle contractions, rhythmic breathing, and pelvic rocking builds up so much more sexual energy and sends it through the entire body. Amazing! The emphasis is on pleasure rather than on orgasm, which ends up being a whole new experience!!!

I also experimented with stimulating different parts of my body. Nipple stimulation, sucking on my fingers. I also tried different dildos—a new experience for me. Betty prefers silicone dildos, but gave me a crystalline acrylic one to try. I quite liked a seven-inch lavender "lover." She also showed me how to stimulate the G spot on the urethra sponge and helped me find different positions to reach it.

Now I meditate and masturbate for forty-five minutes every day. I've been having loving orgasmic times with myself and I have never felt so loved. My orgasms are the best I've ever had. I never could have dreamed this would happen without a partner. It was *so* liberating.

ANNIE SPRINKLE'S SLUTS AND GODDESSES WORKSHOP

Isa is the forty-year-old mother of a seven-year-old son and a long-time women's health activist. She is an herbalist, a registered nurse, and teaches health and sexuality classes for teens and adults. She took Annie Sprinkle's "Sluts and Goddesses" workshop and found that it changed her concept of her sexuality in remarkable ways:

I knew who Annie Sprinkle was, and wanted to meet her, since I'd admired her work as a sex educator and as a performance artist so much. I received a flyer in the mail for a three-day workshop she was offering in upstate New York called "Sluts and Goddesses," and I was intrigued. In the flyer, Annie spoke of sexuality as being a sacred aspect of our existence, and suggested that we would have the opportunity to expand our sexual energy through Tantric breathing techniques, exploring our sexual personas, and through intensive genital massage, learn to experience full-body energy orgasms. I knew I wanted to go. I was just coming out of a long relationship in which I'd felt stifled sexually, and this was not the first time I'd experienced this in partnerships. For many years and with many partners I'd felt that it was not okay for me to express myself sexually as fully as I longed to do. I knew I wanted the experience of having sex that was intensely physical and deeply emotional—I just didn't know how to get there. I also wanted to meet other women who were thinking about and exploring these issues, and who were brave enough to risk exploring and celebrating their sexuality openly. So I drove to upstate in my brother's little MG convertible, giving a ride to another participant, an erotic dancer from the city whom I'd never met. We talked and laughed the whole ride, most of it in an amazing downpour that miraculously ended the moment we arrived at the workshop. We'd been told to bring our sexiest attire, vibrators and lube, jewelry and leather, or whatever else we found sexy. We set up camp on a plateau in the wooded hills, getting ready for we didn't know what yet.

At the first meeting after Annie and her assistants introduced themselves, we formed a circle, and were invited to tell a story about our sexual history. Some women told very funny stories about the first time they kissed or had sex, some women shared wrenching stories of physical abuse or sexual violence: all told stories that we could relate to, and it created an immediate feeling of close bonding and trust. Then we got up and danced together with our eyes closed, to rhythmic music that was deeply sensual and compelling. We danced for ages, on and on, many of us crying or laughing or shouting out, with a heightened awareness of ourselves and each other until we were exhausted. Then we lay down together with our eyes closed, enjoying the tremendous quiet of the early evening. When we got up, Annie told us to dress up in whatever kind of special attire we'd brought, and walk down to the pavilion where she would meet us. She wouldn't tell us anything more except that we were in for a big surprise that night. So we giggled as we made our way back up through the wooded hills to our tents, filled with expectation, and dressed for the evening.

As the sun set we emerged from our tents and walked down the forest path to the pavilion where our meeting would take place. What a sight we must have been traipsing down the mossy path adorned in lacy bras and panties, silk slips, leather vests and straps, or totally naked. At the doorway Annie and her assistants greeted us by smudging fragrant burnt sage on our faces, sprinkling us with rosewater, and whispering sexy messages in our ears. The room had been transformed into a virtual pleasure palace with bolts of dark velvet and satin draped from the ceiling and around the windows and doors. Incense was burning, candles were lit everywhere, and a drummer was playing intensely moving rhythms, creating a wondrously sensuous atmosphere. In fact, it was so seductive, I felt right away that I never wanted to leave. We were invited to sit in a circle, and the drummer began to play and chant songs and we all joined in.

Then Annie opened her trunk and put a huge pile of "slut" attire of all sizes and styles in the middle of the circle: bras, bustiers, teddies, exquisite sequin dresses, slips, stockings, garter belts, dildo straps and dildos, whips, feather boas, and wigs. On the side of the room there were also tables with lots of makeup and jewelry. We were instructed to dress up, creating a slut personae, and asked to take a new name appropriate to our inner "slut." We each had pictures of ourselves taken, which we put together into an amazing collage. Then, one by one, we danced for each other, tucking fake money into the dancer's lingerie, cheering for and appreciating each dancer. I thought this was really extraordinary, because I'm sure if you had asked us, half of the women there would have sworn that they'd never do this, under any circumstances. But on that night, because of the permission we were given, we all did it. When I performed, I loved myself so much for being so sexy and exhibitionist, and felt so full of joy at being able to reveal myself sexually in "public." Most of the women in the group were heterosexual, and it was especially pleasing to watch them being turned on by women's bodies.

Then we put the "slut" clothes away and Annie put out a huge pile of "goddess" attire of all sizes and styles: that were mostly more elegant versions of the slut outfits, and might have been worn by a Botticelli Venus, and handsome leatherwear that would have been appropriate for your basic dominatrix. We chose goddess names to fit our new personas, and had our pictures taken in our new outfits. Inspired by the dominatrixes, we began flirting and playfully whipping each other with scarves, ribbons, belts, and soft cat-o-nine-tails as we danced. This was a revelation to most of the women there who had always believed that S/M play was dangerous or sleazy, but now saw how harmless and titillating it could be. The music had changed from the pounding rhythms of the slut dancing to more ethereal cadences befitting goddesses, and we danced for each other, taking turns one at a time in the center of the circle. I felt so turned on, able finally to claim and exhibit my exuberant sexuality. Then and there I decided that I wanted to replicate this kind of workshop for other women.

The next day we learned a variety of Tantric ecstatic breathing techniques, including the "fire breath," which is designed to build sexual energy in the entire body to the point of explosion. This particular technique was enormously revelatory for me. While doing it, I discovered that orgasm is so much more than just what happens in my clitoris. We did this and other breathing techniques for a very long time, and it was intensely emotional.

After lunch we went to a high plateau in the woods and did exercises designed to maintain the energy from the breathing and increase our sensitivity toward each other. We were tired but it felt good to keep pushing to new emotional heights. In the evening we went back to the pavilion and found that it had been beautifully redecorated for us, with pillows and soft lighting and sensual music. We sat together in pairs, and Annie coached us through a series of Tantric partnering exercises. We breathed together, exchanged sensual touch, all the while gazing directly and deeply into each other's eyes—a Tantric technique used to promote intimacy. Then Annie and her assistants brought in an opulent feast of soft ripe fruit, bowls of melted chocolate and whipped cream and set it down amongst us. While lying together we fed each other and started decorating each other's bodies while we laughed and licked the sweetness off. We lay in an exhausted pile at the end, sharing life stories and thoughts about the evening. Then we trooped over to an outdoor shower and washed each other off.

The next day we moved to a flower-filled deck in the sun to learn genital massage. First, we did some intensive breathing and full-body massage and then focused on the genitals. Annie showed us a series of specific strokes that she has given very descriptive names such as "around the neighborhood" for light strokes from the pubic mound to the anus; "the pussy pet" for gently cupping and warming the vulva with a hand; "rock around the clit clock" for little finger circles around the clitoral glans; "ringing the doorbell" for pressing into the urethral sponge from the abdomen. Then with permission from our partners (and it was fine to choose not to be entered), we were guided in a series of strokes to pleasure the inside of the vagina, including the urethral sponge, vaginal walls, and cervix. For many women this was the first time they'd had the opportunity to really focus on how different areas of the vagina feel. During this time memories of my own sexual abuse came up very powerfully. Previously, my urethral sponge had been so hypersensitive that it was painful to have it touched deeply, but during this safe, guided breathing and touching exercise, something changed for me and opened up, and now all I feel in that area of my vagina is intense pleasure. Annie kept encouraging us to breathe deeply, to keep the energy that was building up in the clitoris flowing to the rest of the body. At this point she led us to do "the Big Draw," a technique that helped intensify and focus the energy. Those of us who wanted to could have vibrators placed against our clitorises, and since we were so sexually charged many women had dramatically intense whole-body orgasms. During the release I felt amazing tidal waves of energy move throughout my entire body and I felt things I had never felt before. For example, my fingertips, which normally I don't focus on at all, felt like incredible energy whorls and I luxuriated in these unexpected sensations. Afterward we all lay on our mats and blankets, many of us gently laughing or crying quietly, releasing all the energy that we'd created over the course of the weekend. After the genital massage session, we spontaneously started sharing our experiences, and it turned out that many of us had a similar sense of feeling released from deeply embedded feelings of shame or apprehension and of being reborn into a new world of sexual discovery and fulfillment, and were amazed at how healing and safe it was to share this with each other.

Over the next year, and with Annie's guidance and support, Isa and two friends established the Sacred Harlots School of Erotic Mysteries in New York City, billing their sessions as "Opening the Gates: A Series of Guided, Ritualized Workshops for Women." (See Resources)

MY EXPERIENCE AT THE BODY ELECTRIC WORKSHOP

One night over dinner, when the conversation between two activists inevitably turned to sex, a friend told me about the Body Electric workshops for women. The workshops, she said, were designed to help women discover their erotic potential through energy enhancement techniques, body-positive exercises, and erotic massage. "I had the best full-body orgasm I ever had," she said unequivocally. I was definitely intrigued (who wouldn't be?) and a few months later, when I was shopping in Eve's Garden (see page 235) I picked up a flyer for an upcoming workshop. Needless to say, I immediately signed up for the two-and-one-half-day seminar entitled "Celebrating the Body Erotic for Women."

I had previously taken Gina Ogden's seminar on sexuality and spirituality, Betty Dodson's advanced seminar for sexuality educators, and Annie Sprinkle's Sluts and Goddesses workshop. I found each of these programs to be enormously empowering in terms of how I felt about women's sexuality in general and my own in particular, and in many different ways.

I escaped from a soggy rush-hour commute into a spacious loft in lower Manhattan. As I took off my shoes and changed into comfortable workout clothes I observed women who were already there stretching, meditating, or moving rhythmically to the ethereal music pulsating in the background. Much of the first evening was devoted to getting acquainted through various movement exercises, "conscious breathing," and sharing information about ourselves and our expectations for the weekend. We had an ideal group of a dozen participants plus the facilitator and three assistants, including heterosexual women and lesbians from ages twenty-three to seventy. Some were in relationships and some were not. As would be expected in any group of women, some were seeking healing from childhood sexual abuse. One lesbian couple came together. Several women had attended other Body Electric workshops, and one who is a sexuality educator remarked, "I'm always helping other people. I do this every year to help myself." Some were seeking spiritual grounding through sexuality (which Body Electric emphasizes), while others were hoping to discover new sensual techniques and ideas for erotic play as ends in themselves. All, however, wanted to access elusive erotic energy and enhance sexual pleasure and/or orgasmic potential. In the opening circle, a number of women mentioned that they didn't feel good about their bodies and were seeking to improve their self-image. The youngest, at twenty-three, said that she came from a very conservative, religious background, and had signed up for the workshop "to be with other women like myself." My heart nearly broke when the eldest participant said, "I've been married for fifty years, and all this time, my husband has been dead from the neck down." I was moved to imagine the courage it must have taken for her to sign up for this workshop.

Most of us breathe just enough to get by, so the ancient Tantric technique of conscious breathing may seem like work at first. We breathed together rhythmically, deep, relaxing breaths, then fast and forceful. We paired off and breathed together, then coached each other. Walking home later that night, I realized that I really did feel lighter, more alert, energetic, and—pardon the cliché—"alive."

One of the goals of the Body Electric workshop is to help women become more comfortable with their bodies, and although this introductory session is "clothing optional," there is no pressure to undress, or participate in any exercise that makes you squeamish. Alex, the facilitator, set an example by removing her shirt during the warm-up, which gave the shy among us "permission" to do the same. There is a place to sit or lie quietly if you choose not to take part in any particular activity.

After warming up and sharing our impressions about the initial session the next morning, Alex divided us into groups of three. We engaged in "reverential disrobing," in which one woman is blindfolded and gently, ever-so-slowly undressed and caressed. Before this exercise began, Alex made it clear that no one was required to remove any of their clothes, and that we should ask each woman if there was something that she didn't want removed. I really liked this part. It took about fifteen minutes from start to finish, and as each piece of clothing was languidly peeled away, I felt a sense of elation rather than shame or fear. Undressed, we stood in a circle and looked at our bodies, tall or short, lean or voluptuous, and breathed contentment. Then, the tempo of the music increased and we moved from stretching and "shaking out" to ecstatic dancing.

Alex led us through a long, intense breathing exercise that ended in the "Big Draw," the Tantric technique that is used to focus and intensify sexual energy. After lunch, we gathered in a circle around Alex as she performed genital self-examination, describing each visible part of the clitoris or *yoni* (Hindu for genitals) and the many other genital structures that are underneath the skin. Then we sat in a circle and each performed a genital self-examination in turn, talking about how we felt about our genitals and how our concept of them had evolved over time. This was by turns heartwarming, funny, and poignant as we described how we had thought about the unnamed structures "down there" as children and what we called them.

Then, two experienced assistants demonstrated nurturing massage using cornstarch rather than massage oil, which allows for a feather-light touch. Afterward, we broke into groups of three and performed massages on each other. Surprisingly, the cornstarch felt like cool raindrops as it was sprinkled on, and it made our skin feel miraculously silky. Having four hands glide over your body with varying pressure and a touch is definitely a deluxe sensuous experience. We all ended up enormously relaxed and looking like powdered doughnuts. That night, I could barely make it home before I collapsed, not from exhaustion but from being completely unwound, as if the normal tensions that hold body and soul together had been loosened. I fell into a deep sleep hours before my normal bedtime.

Looking around the circle at the faces and bodies on Sunday morning, I felt as if we had been together for much longer than a dozen hours. We discussed how the first two days had gone for us. Two of Alex's assistants then demonstrated full-body erotic and genital massage, emphasizing communication between the giver and the receiver, to ensure that the receiver is getting the kind of strokes and stimulation that she likes, and that the giver does nothing that is unwanted. The givers wore latex gloves for genital touching, and the receiver was encouraged to use her vibrator if she wished.

The erotic massage ritual is the centerpiece of the Body Erotic workshop and is quite literally the climax of the weekend. From the opening circle, the movement, breathing exercises, nudity, genital exploration, and sharing information about our sexuality progressively increase in intensity and are carefully designed to promote intimacy, banish sexual shame, and build energy and anticipation. When my turn came, I lay blindfolded on a massage table as every part of my body was pressed, caressed, soothed, fanned with cool breaths, and vibrated. To my surprise, I found the head massage very exquisite. It seemed to make my hair follicles come alive and gave me shivers up and down my spine. I also *re*discovered that the little indentation at the base of the throat between the clavicle bones (the spot Ralph Fiennes adored on Kristin Scott Thomas's neck in *The English Patient*) is one of my most hypersensitive spots.

When sexual activity is primarily or exclusively genitally focused, the sensory input travels up the spinal cord to the brain and back. In full-body erotic massage, the genitals are the sacred focal point that everything feeds into, and, whether or not orgasm occurs, the energy seems to be readily reflected not just up and down the spine but to distant body parts as well. I felt as if I was being massaged by the eight-armed Hindu goddess, one hand caressing my temples while another kneaded my tummy, another tugging on my nipples, fingers of a different hand on my clitoris, and another lightly tickling my feet. When I felt ready, I reached for my vibrator and began having one orgasm after another—and entered a state I can only describe as "orgasmic nirvana."

The sounds of sex are unlike any other. They may at first be mistaken for cries of pain, but there are always throaty overtones of other-worldly pleasure. Then you hear openmouthed howls, squeals of rapture, giggles of delight, and eventually whimpers of surrender. All around me, I heard the sounds of women in ecstasy and I added my own voice to this extraordinary cacophony.

As late afternoon clouds rolled in over the Hudson, we basked in the afterglow of our individual experiences. In the closing circle, we thanked Alex by moving in and placing our hands on her body. We sat quietly in a final moment of meditation, when a stunning thunderclap burst nearby, echoing through the concrete canyons of Tribeca, rattling the window panes, and sending vibrations through us all. In unison we burst into cheers of delight at this uncanny cosmic comment on our erotic adventure.

WORKSHOPS GALORE
A Little Something for Everyone

Experiential workshops like Dodson's, Sprinkle's, and the Body Electric School are just a few of the many programs from a wide variety of perspectives designed to enable women and their partners to enhance their sexual experiences in a safe, supportive environment. Sprinkle continues to do her Sluts and Goddesses workshop in the San Francisco Bay area and the northeast. She also has a video version. Dodson no longer teaches her Bodysex sessions, but her program and individual sex coaching sessions are also on video. Alex Jade, who led the Body Electric class that I took, also teaches "Cunt Classes," a workshop intended to help women explore issues such as anatomy and female ejaculation, as well as vaginal and anal eroticism, in much greater depth. Ronnie, one of Alex's students, told me:

> I had taken a Body Electric workshop and it was so transforming for me. It helped lower my inhibitions about trying anything new and exploring my erotic potential, and that was so positive that I wanted to go farther. I found that Cunt Class provided the most amazing sense of discovery and liberation. The level of detail was so revealing! I had never ejaculated before, but it was so exciting to learn that I had the potential

to, and I learned other things that I never came across in health classes or even in my own reading.

The famous Good Vibrations sex boutique has picked up its toys and taken to the road. This ever inventive group offers an impressive roster of workshops that they stage around California, occasional remote spots in the United States, and even in Mexico (in Spanish yet)! Their repertoire includes workshops on masturbation, improving sexual self-image, sex toys, "lesbian blue movies," and sexuality and spirituality.

Kim Airs, proprietor of Boston's woman-oriented sex boutique, Grand Opening!, teaches a variety of workshops covering everything from female ejaculation to anal sex. Kim even has a workshop entitled "Zaftig! Sex and Sensuality for the Well-Rounded Woman." The boutique's most popular class is "Stripping for Women." For those who want to see the real thing, she conducts a field visit to a well-known local stripping emporium. She also offers an innovative workshop for men on pleasuring women, including information on women's anatomy and tips regarding sex toys and activities designed to enhance and enliven sex.

There are literally hundreds of instructors who teach Tantric spiritual and sexual practices around the United States, Europe, and Asia. Several have crossed over into the mainstream by writing books and ng workshops that emphasize the erotic aspects of Tantra ng with traditional ceremonies and rituals. One of the best known of these is the Sky Dancing Tantra International, founded by Margo Anand, whose books, *The Art of Sexual Ecstasy* and *The Art of Sexual Magic,* have become classics in the field. Margo and her colleagues teach an "Ecstasy Workshop," utilizing a variety of Tantric techniques to help participants experience "high sex." This workshop is also available on video (see Resources).

Mantak and Maneewan Chia are undoubtedly the best known teachers of Taoist spiritual traditions, and their books *Cultivating Female Sexual Energy* and *Cultivating Male Sexual Energy* lay out the basis of Taoist sexual practices. Recently, Mantak Chia took a bold step into the mainstream when he wrote *The Multi-Orgasmic Man* with Douglas Abrams Arava. The book describes the age-old technique of ejaculatory control in detail and should be useful to any man who wants to learn this technique. Those interested in learning "Sexual Kung Fu" (Taoist sexual practices) can check Chia's Web site (see Resources).

SEX IN THE TWENTY-FIRST CENTURY

Sex in this new age has the potential to become more egalitarian, user-friendly, exciting, and physically and psychologically rewarding than it has ever been. I see more and more women assertively exploring their sexuality, discovering what feels good and just how good it can feel. I watch as the antimasturbation lobby goes down in flaming defeat. As women articulate their sexual desires, I bear witness to more and better erotica being published and filmed. I also see the crumbling of the heterosexual "norm" and increasing acceptance of "ambisexuality." I see an increasing number of men willing to learn ejaculatory control for their partners' pleasure as well as their own, and many women discovering their ability to have multiple orgasms, teaching their partners how to make this possible. I also see many women and men having ecstatic sex with or without male erections, even without orgasms, and feeling that it is "real," physically rewarding, and life affirming.

GLOSSARY

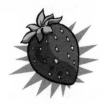

anal sphincter (SFINGK-ter) **muscle**: The muscle that encircles the anus and opens and closes to allow the passage of feces. In addition to maintaining fecal continence, this muscle can be consciously relaxed to allow the passage of a finger, penis, or sex toy for sexual pleasure. Strands of this muscle are woven into the bulbocavernosus muscle and together they form a figure eight.

body of caverns: One of two types of erectile tissue in the clitoris composed primarily of tightly packed arteries. The clitoral bulbs are composed of cavernous erectile tissue. During sexual response, the arteries fill with blood, which becomes trapped and is released by orgasm, or, if no orgasm occurs, it seeps out over a period of hours.

bridle: The point beneath the glans of the clitoris where the inner edges of the inner lips meet, forming an upside-down V. The Latin term is frenulum.

bulbocavernosus (bul-bo-kav-er-NO-sus) **muscle**, or BC muscle: Twin muscles lying underneath the outer lips and on top of the bulbs of the clitoris. The BC muscle is attached to the perineal sponge, the bulbs, and the suspensory ligament of the clitoris.

bulbs: Twin erectile structures of the clitoris, shaped somewhat like miniature eggplants and composed of densely packed and folded arteries and veins, a type of erectile tissue called corpus cavernosum, or cavernous body. During sexual response, the bulbs fill with blood, which becomes trapped and is released by the spasms of orgasm. If no orgasm occurs, the blood will seep out over a few hours.

clitoris (KLIT-er-ris): The genital organ of women that includes erectile tissue, glands, muscles and ligaments, nerves, and blood vessels. Although structures are arranged differently, the clitoris is entirely equivalent to the penis.

corpus cavernosum (COR-pus-kav-er-NO-sum): See *body of caverns*.

corpus spongiosum (COR-pus spun-gee-O-sum): See *spongy body*.

consensual role playing (CRP): A sexual game in which both partners or all members of a group establish and agree to rules and set limits of erotically stimulating scenarios, including exhibitionism, voyeurism, dominance and submission (D&S), and sadomasochism (S/M). Conscientious practitioners of CRP insist on three essential elements: (1) Safe: that the players always abide by safer sex guidelines, that no activity will provide more pain than has been agreed upon, endanger vital organs, or inflict any permanent damage; (2) Sane: that limits for both physical and psychological pain are agreed upon and respected; (3) Consensual: that both or all partners voluntarily and knowingly agree to the terms of sex play and games.

crura (KROO ra): See *legs*.

dominance and submission (D&S): Sexual activities in which one person plays a dominant or controlling role, and the other plays a submissive role. Most practitioners tend to prefer one role over the other, but some enjoy both roles.

egg tubes: The twin egg transport tubes. One end of each tube is attached to the uterus and the other open ends float near the ovaries. At ovulation, the wavy fingers (fembria) of the tubes capture the egg, which has popped through the ovarian wall, and with an undulating movement (peristalsis), move the egg through the tube into the uterus. Fertilization usually occurs in the outer quarter of the tube several days after ovulation. Also known as Fallopian tubes.

erection: Filling of the erectile tissues of the clitoris or penis during sexual response. The blood becomes trapped by vasocongestion until the blood is released by orgasm or it seeps out over a few hours.

exhibitionism (ek-se-BISH-en-iz-mm): Performing sexually for the benefit of one's self and/or others. Exhibitionist activities include talking, dressing up, or acting out fantasies with a partner or before an audience.

Fallopian (fa-LO-pee-an) **tubes**: See *egg tubes*.

female ejaculation: The spurt, squirt, gush, or dribble of an alkaline fluid that is manufactured in up to three dozen or more tiny prostatic glands embedded in the spongy erectile tissue surrounding the female urethra. This fluid is directly equivalent to the alkaline secretion of the male prostate.

female prostate: Up to three dozen or more tiny glands embedded in the urethral sponge, which produce an alkaline secretion during sexual response. Some of these glands, referred to as periurethral glands, empty directly into the urethra. Two larger glands located near the urethral opening, referred to as the paraurethral glands, empty through the paraurethral ducts on either side of the urethral opening.

fork: A short band of mucous membrane formed where the lower ends of the inner lips of the clitoris meet just beneath the vaginal opening. The medical term is fourchette, meaning "little fork."

fourchette (foor-SHET): See *fork*.

frenulum (FREN-u-lum): See *bridle*.

front commissure (KOM-I-sur): The point above the glans where the outer edges of the inner lips meet and form the clitoral hood. This junction marks the upper extent of the visible portions of the clitoris. Also called the anterior (meaning "front") commissure.

genitals (JEN-I-tals): The organs of reproduction. In women, these include the ovaries, egg tubes, uterus and its neck, or cervix, and vagina. The male reproductive organ is much more complex, and includes all of the sexual structures as well.

glans (GLANZ): The head or tip of the clitoris. Richly endowed with nerve endings, the sole purpose of the glans is to produce pleasurable sensations.

hood: The crinkled fold of skin formed by the outer edges of the inner lips that covers the glans of the clitoris and is directly equivalent to the male foreskin.

homologous (ho-MOL-e-gus): Organs or body parts that correspond in structure and origin. The clitoris is often said to be homologous to the penis, but many definitions characterize it as a miniature homolog.

hymen (HI-men): A fold of mucous membrane that partially covers the vaginal opening. The hymen may be torn during normal childhood activities or during first intercourse. In the past, an unbroken hymen was thought to be proof of virginity, but given the essential fragility of this tissue, it is no longer considered a reliable indicator.

inner lips: Two parallel, highly sensitive folds of skin that enclose the urethral and vaginal openings, forming the introitus. The outer edges of the inner lips meet above the glans to form the clitoral hood and the inner edges meet beneath the glans forming the bridle. Called labia minora (little lips) in Latin.

introitus (in-TROI-tus): The space formed by the inner lips that encloses the urethral and vaginal openings.

ischiocavernosus (IS-ke-o-KA-ver-NO-sus) **muscles** (IC muscles): Twin strips of muscle attached to the clitoral legs that flare out as if to form the sides of a triangle. The other ends are attached to the ischium bones (the bones we sit on). The IC muscles help erection by compressing erectile tissues and trapping blood in them.

Kegel (KAY-gul) **exercises**: Named after Dr. Arnold Kegel, the gynecologist who developed this exercise in the 1940s, these exercises are designed to strengthen the pubococcygeus (PC) and levator ani muscles, which support the pelvic organs to maintain continence and produce orgasm.

legs: Two slightly bowed arcs of spongy erectile tissue that originate where the shaft, or body, of the clitoris divides. The legs bow slightly as they separate from the shaft, like the wishbone of a chicken. The Latin term is *crura*.

levator ani (le-VA-tur AN-ee) **muscle** (LA muscle): See *pubococcygeus* muscle.

meatus (me-A-tus): An opening or passage. The urethral meatus is located in the introitus, just above the vaginal opening.

mons veneris (mons ve-NER-is): See *pubic mound.*

Mound of Venus: See *pubic mound.*

orgasm: Pleasurable spasms of the clitoral muscles and release of sexual chemicals that result from an overload of stimulation. The spasms of orgasm flush blood from the erectile tissues.

outer lips: Twin pads of fatty tissue enfolding the visible portions of the clitoris. The commonly used Latin term is labia majora, meaning "large lips."

oxytocin (ok-see-TO-sin): A hormone manufactured by the pituitary gland that promotes labor during childbirth and stimulates the release of milk for breast feeding. Oxytocin is also released during sexual stimulation of the breasts and increases sensitivity and engorgement of the genitals.

paraurethral (pa-ra-u-REE-thral) **glands**: Female prostatic glands located near the urethral opening, which empty through two paraurethral ducts that are usually located at four o'clock and eight o'clock adjacent to the opening. Also called Skene's glands.

pelvic floor muscle exercises: See *Kegel exercises*.

pelvic floor muscles: The pubococcygeus (PC) and the levator ani (LA) muscles, which form the pelvic floor. These muscles stretch from the pubic bone to the tailbone (coccyx) forming a sling or hammock to support the uterus and bladder. The urethra and vagina pass through these muscles. They also constrict the bulbs of the clitoris, helping to maintain erection, and spasm, contributing to orgasm.

perineal (per-I-NEE-al) **sponge**: A densely packed, tangled mass of blood vessels underneath the perineum that becomes engorged with blood during sexual response and is consequently highly sensitive to pressure and vibration. Sometimes referred to as the perineal body.

perineum (per-I-NEE-um): The short bridge of skin that separates the visible portions of the vagina from the anus. The perineal sponge lies just beneath the perineum.

prostate (PRA-state) **gland**: In men, the fibrous, muscular, glandular structure about the size of a walnut that is located just below the bladder, which surrounds the urethra and produces an alkaline secretion that is squeezed into the semen as it passes through the urethra. The prostatic secretion is composed of enzymes, calcium, zinc, and other substances and makes up about 15 percent of the male ejaculate.

prostatic acid phosphatase (pra-STAT-ic-A-sid FOS-fa-taze) (PAP): An enzyme manufactured by the male prostate, and found in high levels in secretions from the female prostate.

prostate specific antigen (PSA): A protein produced by the prostate that is attached to cells to identify them as specifically made by the prostate.

pubic mound: The hairy, fatty pad of tissue that lies above the pubic bone between the abdomen and the clitoris. Also called *mons veneris* or Mound of Venus.

pubococcygeus (PU-bo-cox-e-GEE-us) **muscle** (PC muscle): Another name for the levator ani, the part of the pelvic diaphragm, the broad, flat sheet of muscle that forms the bottom of the pelvic floor. During sexual response, the PC muscle contracts, contributing to erection by compressing the erectile tissues of the clitoris. In concert with other clitoral muscles, the PC muscle spasms during orgasm, forcing blood out of erectile tissues, and creating pleasurable sensations. The PC muscle is also critical in supporting the bladder and uterus.

pudendum (pu-DEN-dum): A Latin word meaning "shame." The plural, pudenda, refers collectively to the female genital organ, although originally, it referred to both the female and male genitals.

round ligament: The ends of these twin ligaments are attached to the uterus near the beginning of the egg tubes, and the other ends are woven into the soft tissue underneath each of the outer lips.

sadomasochism (SA-do-MAS-e-kiz-em) (S/M): Sexual or other activity in which one person dominates or inflicts pain on another. See dominance and submission.

shaft: The short segment of spongy erectile tissue that is attached to the glans of the clitoris on one end, and folds and divides on the other to form the legs. Also called the body of the clitoris.

Skene's glands: See *paraurethral glands*.

spongy body (*corpus spongiosum*): One of two types of erectile tissue in the clitoris that is composed of tightly packed arteries, veins, and fibrous connective tissue. The glans, shaft, legs, and urethral sponge of the clitoris are composed of spongy body.

suspensory (su-SPEN-so-ree) **ligament**: The ends of these twin ligaments are attached to the ovaries. The other ends converge and are attached to the glans of the clitoris. During sexual response, these ligaments tighten, pulling the glans back underneath the hood.

Tantra (TAN-tra): The mystical Hindu philosophy emphasizing the interconnectedness of humans with the natural world and the quest for understanding the multifaceted mysteries of existence. Sex is considered to be the central sacrament of Tantra and the most direct pathway in the quest for knowledge of the divine.

Taoism (DOW-iz-um): The ancient Chinese philosophical system that emphasizes sex as the most reliable way to discover the Tao (the path or way) to enlightenment about the meaning of life and humanity's relationship to the universe.

transverse perineal (per-i-NEE-al) **muscle** (TP muscle): This tight band of muscle forms the base of the triangle formed on each side by the ischiocavernosus (IC) muscles. At its midpoint, the TP muscle is woven into the perineal sponge.

urethra (u-REE-thra): The canal through which urine is emptied.

urethral (u-REE-thral) **opening**: The opening thorough which urine empties from the body, located between the glans of the clitoris and the vaginal opening.

urethral (u-REE-thral) **sponge**: The spongy erectile tissue that surrounds the urethra in both the clitoris and the penis. Many tiny glands hidden in the convoluted folds of the sponge produce an alkaline fluid similar to that produced by the male prostate.

urine (UR-in): The liquid waste product manufactured by the kidneys and stored in the bladder. Urine is 95 percent water and 5 percent organic matter.

urogenital diaphragm (u-ro-JEN-I-tal-DI-a-fram): The flat, triangular-shaped muscle that underlies the triangle formed by the ischiocavernosus muscles and the transverse perineal muscle.

vagina (va-GI-na): The mucous membrane-lined passage between the cervix, the lower tip of the uterus, and the outside of the body. The vagina has few nerve endings and is not actively involved in sexual response. The outer third of the vagina is surrounded by clitoral structures and muscles. The vagina's primary function is reproductive. It collects semen, serves as a conduit for menstrual blood and, during childbirth, as the birth canal.

vasocongestion (VA-so-con-JES-chun): The temporary or chronic accumulation of blood in an organ or body part. During sexual response blood floods into the erectile tissues of the clitoris, resulting in vasocongestion. The blood is then flushed by orgasm or seeps out over a few hours. If the blood is not adequately flushed, some women experience a feeling of fullness in the genitals. This feeling may be relieved by masturbation or sexual activity with a partner. In the past, women who had few if any rewarding sexual outlets may have experienced chronic vasocongestion. This condition was termed "hysteria," and was often relieved by secret masturbation or by a midwife or doctor.

vestibule (VES-ti-bul): A passage or antechamber. This is the space created by the inner lips that begins at the bridle underneath the glans of the clitoris and ends at the fork below the vaginal opening, enfolding the urethral and vaginal openings. Although the vestibule is created by clitoral structures, since it is just a space it is not considered to be a feature of the clitoris.

virginity (vir-GIN-I-tee): In the past, when sex was defined through its reproductive function, virginity meant that a woman had never experienced intercourse. Today, the meaning of sex has expanded to include any type of activity or stimulation that is sexually pleasurable, and the concept of virginity is rendered meaningless.

voyeurism (voi-YUR-iz-em): The practice of obtaining or enhancing sexual stimulation by watching the sexual performance of another person, either with his or her consent, or secretly. Watching erotic movies alone or with others could also be considered voyeuristic.

vulva: The vulva is variously defined, but the essential meaning of the word is "covering." Often, definitions of vulva include most of the visible structures of the clitoris and even occasionally the bulbs, but this definition evolved in the absence of a complete definition of the clitoris. The vulva correctly includes the pubic mound and the outer lips.

vulvovaginal (vul-vo-VAJ-I-nal) **glands**: Two small glands located beneath the vaginal opening. These glands produce a small amount of viscous mucous during sexual response, which helps to lubricate the vaginal opening. Also called Bartholin's glands.

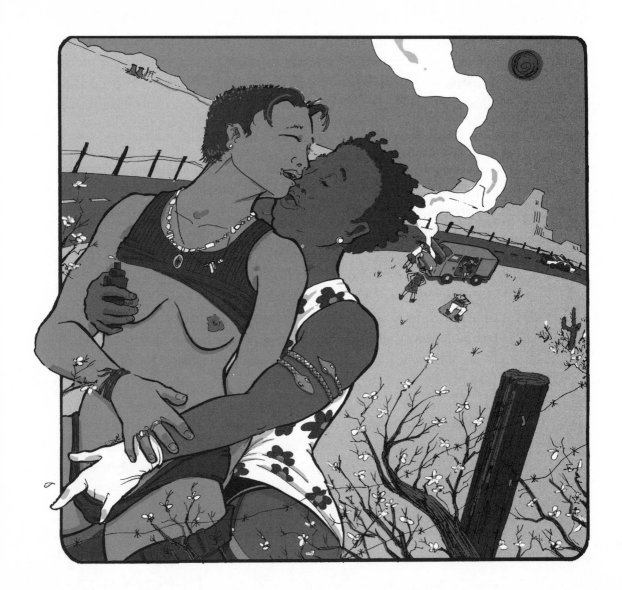

RESOURCES

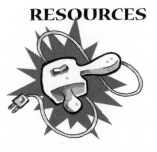

In the last decade, there has been an explosion of books on every aspect of sexuality and, thanks to the proliferation of online booksellers, such books are almost universally available for purchase. To include more than a representative selection would be a book in itself, so I am listing books that I found interesting or that informed my understanding of sexuality in one way or another. For a wider selection of topics and points of view, check out my suggestions at the end of each section, the numerous Web sites, as well as the online booksellers. For a concentrated library of lesbian works, refer to the Naiad Press catalog and Web site.

NONFICTION

Anatomy of Love: The Natural History of Monogamy, Adultery, and Divorce, Helen Fisher (W.W. Norton, 1992).

Annie Sprinkle: Post-Pòrn Modernist, Annie Sprinkle (Cleis Press, 1998).

Beyond Definition: New Writing from Gay and Lesbian San Francisco, Marci Blackman and Trebor Healey, eds. (Manic D Press, 1994).

Bi Any Other Name: Bisexual People Speak Out, Loraine Hutchins and Lani Kaahumanu, eds. (Alyson Publications, 1990).

Boston Marriages: Romantic but Asexual Relationships Among Contemporary Lesbians, Esther D. Rothblum and Kathleen A. Brehony, eds. (University of Massachusetts Press, 1993).

Changing Bodies, Changing Lives: A Book for Teens on Sex and Relationships, Ruth Bell (Times Books, 1998).

Couples, Sex, and Power: The Politics of Desire, S. Dallos and R. Dallos (Open University Press, 1997).

Defending Pornography: Free Speech, Sex, and the Fight for Women's Rights, Nadine Strossen (Scribner, 1995).

Different Loving: The World of Sexual Dominance and Submission, Gloria G. Brame, William D. Brame, and Jon Jacobs, eds. (Villard, 1996).

Disorders of Desire: Sex and Gender in Modern American Sexology, Janice M. Irvine (Temple University Press, 1990).

Dyke Life: From Growing Up to Growing Old, a Celebration of the Lesbian Experience, Karla Jay (Basic Books, 1997).

The Erotic Impulse: Honoring the Sensual Self, David Steinberg, ed. (Tarcher, 1992).

ESO (Extended Sexual Orgasm), Alan P. Brauer and Donna J. Brauer (Time Warner, 1983).

ESO Workbook, Alan P. Brauer and Donna J. Brauer (Time Warner, 1983).

Eve's Secrets: A New Theory of Female Sexuality, Josephine Lowndes Sevely (Random House, 1987).

Femalia, Joani Blank, ed. (Down There Press, 1993).

Feminism and Sexuality: A Reader, Stevi Jackson and Sue Scott, eds. (Columbia University Press, 1996).

Forbidden Flowers: More Women's Sexual Fantasies, Nancy Friday (Pocket, 1993).

Full Exposure: Opening Up to Your Sexual Creativity and Erotic Expression, Susie Bright (HarperSan Francisco, 1999).

Getting It On: A Condom Reader, Mitch Roberson and Julie Dubner (Soho Press, 1999).

Going All the Way: Teenage Girls' Tales of Sex, Romance, and Pregnancy, Sharon Thompson (Hill and Wang, 1995).

Hearts of Men: American Dreams and the Flight from Commitment, Barbara Ehrenreich (Anchor, 1984).

Heterosexual Politics, Mary Maynard and June Purvis, eds. (Taylor & Francis, 1995).

The Hite Report on Male Sexuality, Shere Hite (Ballantine, 1981).

The Hite Report on the Family: Growing Up Under the Patriarchy, Shere Hite (Grove Press, 1994).

The Hite Report: A Nationwide Study of Female Sexuality, Shere Hite (Dell, 1976).

How to Persuade Your Lover to Use a Condom… And Why You Should, Patti Breitman, Kim Knutson, and Paul Reed (Prima Publishing, 1994).

Intimate Matters: A History of Sexuality in America, John D'Emilio and Estelle B. Freedman (University of Chicago Press, 1997).

Lesbian Erotics, Karla Jay, ed. (New York University Press, 1995).

The Lesbian Love Companion, Marny Hall (HarperSanFrancisco, 1998).

Lesbian Sex: An Oral History, Susan Johnson (Naiad Press, 1997).

Making Sex: Body and Gender from the Greeks to Freud, Thomas Laqueur (Harvard University Press, 1990).

The Mismeasure of Woman: Why Women are Not the Better Sex, the Inferior Sex, or the Opposite Sex, Carol Tavris, (Touchstone, 1992).

My Enemy, My Love: Women, Men, and the Dilemmas of Gender, Janice Levine (Anchor/Doubleday, 1993).

My Secret Garden: Women's Sexual Fantasies, Nancy Friday (Pocket, 1998).

The Mythology of Sex: An Illustrated Exploration of Sexual Customs and Practices from Ancient Times to the Present, Sarah Dening (Macmillan, 1996).

A New View of a Woman's Body, The Federation of Feminist Women's Health Centers (Feminist Health Press, 1991).

Nymphomania: A History, Carol Groneman (W. W. Norton, 2000).

Pleasure and Danger: Exploring Female Sexuality, Carole S. Vance, ed. (Routledge, 1995).

Powers of Desire: The Politics of Sexuality, Ann Snitow, C. Stansell, and Sharon Thompson (Monthly Review Press, 1983).

The Prehistory of Sex: Four Million Years of Human Sexual Culture, Timothy Taylor (Bantam Books, 1997).

Queer Looks: Perspectives on Lesbian and Gay Film and Video, Martha Gever, Pratibha Parmar, and John Greyson, eds. (Routledge, 1993).

The Reign of the Phallus: Sexual Politics in Ancient Athens, Eva C. Keuls (University of California Press, 1985).

Re-Making Love: The Feminization of Sex, Barbara Ehrenreich, Elizabeth Hess, and Gloria Jacobs (Anchor, 1986).

Sacred Pleasure: Sex, Myth, and the Politics of the Body—New Paths to Power and Love, Riane Eisler (HarperCollins, 1996).

Sex and Sensibility: Reflections on Forbidden Mirrors and the Will to Censor, Marcia Pally (Ecco Press, 1994).

Sex Exposed: Sexuality and the Pornography Debate, Lynn Segal and Mary McIntosh (Virago Press, 1992).

Sex for One: The Joy of Self-Loving, Betty Dodson (Crown, 1987).

Sex Is Not a Natural Act and Other Essays, Leonore Tiefer (Westview Press, 1995).

Sex, Power and Pleasure, M. Valverde (The Women's Press, 1985).

Sex: Real People Talk About What They Really Do, Harry Maurer (Penguin, 1994).

Sex: The Most Fun You Can Have Without Laughing and Other Quotations, William Cole and Louis Phillips, eds. (St. Martin's Press, 1990).

Sex Variant Women in Literature, Jeanette H. Foster (Naiad Press, 1985).

Sexing the Millennium: Women and the Sexual Revolution, Linda Grant (Grove Press, 1994).

Sexual Salvation: Affirming Women's Sexual Rights and Pleasures, Naomi McCormick (Praeger, 1994).

Slut! Growing Up Female with a Bad Reputation, Leora Tanenbaum (Seven Stories Press, 1999).

Straight Sex: Rethinking the Politics of Pleasure, Lynne Segal (University of California Press, 1994).

Susie Bright's Sexual Reality: A Virtual Sex World Reader, Susie Bright (Cleis Press, 1992).

Susie Bright's Sexual State of the Union, Susie Bright (Simon & Schuster, 1997).

Susie Bright's Sexwise, Susie Bright (Cleis Press, 1995).

Susie Sexpert's Lesbian Sex World, Susie Bright (Cleis Press, 1990).

in: *Talking About Sex, Class & Literature*, Dorothy Allison (Firebrand Books, 1994).

Talk Dirty to Me: An Intimate Philosophy of Sex, Sallie Tisdale (Doubleday, 1994).

The Technology of Orgasm: "Hysteria," the Vibrator, and Women's Sexual Satisfaction, Rachel P. Maines (Johns Hopkins University Press, 1999).

A Time of Our Lives: Women Write on Sex After 40, Dena Taylor and Amber Sumrall, eds. (Crossing Press, 1993).

Woman: An Intimate Geography, Natalie Angier (Houghton Mifflin, 1999).

Women and Love: A Cultural Revolution in Progress, Shere Hite (Knopf, 1987).

Women on Sex: Women of All Ages Talk Intimately About Every Aspect of Their Sexual Experiences, Susan Quilliam (Barricade Books, 1994).

Women on Top: How Real Life Has Changed Women's Sexual Fantasies, Nancy Friday (Pocket Books, 1991).

Women, Passion and Celibacy, S. Cline, Carol Southern Books, 1993.

Women Who Love Sex: An Inquiry into the Expanding Spirit of Women's Erotic Experience, Gina Ogden, (Womanspirit Press, 1999).

Women's Sexuality Across the Life Span: Challenging Myths, Creating Meanings, Judith C. Daniluk (Guilford Press, 1998).

FICTION

Best American Erotica 1994, 1995, 1996, 1997, 1999, and *2000*, Susie Bright, ed. (Touchstone, 1994, 1995, 1996, 1997, 1999, 2000).

By Word of Mouth: Lesbians Write the Erotic, Lee Fleming, ed. (Gynergy Books, 1989).

Deep Down: New Sensual Writing by Women, Laura Chester, ed. (Faber & Faber, 1989).

The Erotic Edge: 22 Erotic Stories for Couples, Lonnie Garfield Barbach (Plume, 1996).

Erotic Interludes: Tales Told by Women, Lonnie Barbach, ed. (Penguin,1995).

The Erotic Naiad, Katherine V. Forrest and Barbara Grier, eds. (Naiad Press, 1992).

Erotique Noire/Black Erotica, Miriam Decosta-Willis, Reginald Martinm, and Roseann P. Bell, eds. (Anchor, 1993).

Fever: Sensual Stories by Women Writers, Michele Slung, ed. (Harper-Collins, 1995).

Herotica: Erotic Short Stories about Women's Desire, Susie Bright, ed. (Passion Press, 1995).

Herotica 2: A Collection of Women's Erotic Fiction, Susie Bright and Joanie Blank, eds. (Plume, 1992).

Herotica 3: A Collection of Women's Erotic Fiction, Susie Bright, ed. (Plume, 1994).

Herotica 4: A New Collection of Erotic Writing by Women, Marcy Sheiner, ed. (Plume, 1996).

Herotica 5: A New Collection of Women's Erotic Fiction, Marcie Sheiner, ed. (Plume, 1998).

Herotica 6: A New Collection of Women's Erotica, Marcy Sheiner, ed. (Plume, 1999).

The Key to Everything: Classic Lesbian Love Poems, Gerry Gomez Pearlberg, ed. (St. Martin's Press, 1995).

The Literary Lover: Great Stories of Passion and Romance, Larry Dark, ed. (Penguin, 1993).

The Mammoth Book of Erotica, Maxim Jakubowski, ed. (Carroll & Graf, 1994).

Pandora's Box 2: An Anthology of Erotic Writing by Women (Black Lace Series), Kerri Sharp, ed. (London Bridge, 1998).

Pandora's Box 3: An Anthology of Erotic Writing by Women (Black Lace Series); Kerri Sharp, ed. (Virgin, 1998).

The Penguin Book of Erotic Stories by Women, Richard Glyn Jones and A. Susan Williams, eds. (Viking/Penguin, 1995).

Pleasures, Robbi Somers (Naiad Press, 1989).

Pleasures: Women Write Erotica, Lonnie Barbach, ed. (Harper & Row, 1984).

The Second Coming: A Leatherdyke Reader, Pat Claifia and Robin Sweeney, eds. (Alyson Publications, 1996).

Sex Toy Tales, Anne Semans and Cathy Winks, eds. (Down There Press, 1988).

The Sexually Dominant Woman: A Workbook for Nervous Beginners, Lady Green (Greenery Press, 1998).

Slow Hand, Michelle Slung, ed. (HarperPerennial, 1992).

XXXOOO: Love and Kisses from Annie Sprinkle (Thirty post-porn postcards), Katherine Gates and Camille Adams, eds. (Cleis Press, 1998).

SEX ADVICE

Ask Me Anything: A Sex Therapist Answers the Most Important Questions for the '90s, Marty Klein (Simon & Schuster, 1992).

Becoming Orgasmic: A Sexual and Personal Growth Program for Women, Julia Heiman and Joseph LoPiccolo (Simon & Schuster, 1988).

Come Play With Me: Games and Toys for Creative Lovers, Joan Elizabeth Lloyd (Warner Books, 1994).

Exhibitionism for the Shy: Show Off, Dress Up, and Talk Hot, Carol Queen. (Down There Press, 1995).

For Each Other: Sharing Sexual Intimacy, Lonnie Garfield Barbach (Signet, 1984).

For Yourself: The Fulfillment of Female Sexuality, Lonnie Barbach (New American Library, 1991).

Going the Distance: Finding and Keeping Lifelong Love, Lonnie Barbach and David L. Geisinger (Plume, 1993).

The Good Vibrations Guide to Sex, Cathy Winks and Anne Semans (Cleis Press, 1994).

The Good Vibrations Guide to the G Spot, Cathy Winks (Down There Press, 1998).

Good Vibrations: The Complete Guide to Vibrators, Joani Blank (Down There Press, 1982).

Great Sex Weekend: A 48-Hour Guide to Rekindling Sparks for Bold, Busy, or Bored Lovers: Includes 24-Hour Plans for the Really Busy, Pepper Schwartz, Ph.D, and Janet Lever, Ph.D (Putnam, 1998).

The Kinsey Institute New Report on Sex, June M. Reinisch with Ruth Beasley (St. Martin's Press, 1990).

Lesbian Passion, JoAnn Loulan (Spinsters Ink, 1987).

Lesbian Sex, JoAnn Loulan (Spinsters Ink, 1984).

The Lesbian Sex Book, Wendy Caster (Alyson, 1993).

Let Me Count the Ways: Discovering Great Sex Without Intercourse, Marty Klein (Tarcher, 1999).

The Multi-Orgasmic Man: How Any Man Can Experience Multiple Orgasms and Dramatically Enhance His Sexual Relationship, Mantak Chia and Douglas Abrams Arava (HarperSan Francisco, 1996).

Ordinary Women, Extraordinary Sex: Releasing the Passion Within, Sandra Scantling and Sue Browder (Dutton, 1993).

Sapphistry: The Book of Lesbian Sexuality, Pat Califia (Naiad Press, 1988).

Sexual Pleasure: Reaching New Heights of Sexual Arousal and Intimacy, Barbara Keesling (Hunter House, 1993).

Turn Ons: Pleasing Yourself While You Please Your Lover, Lonnie Garfield Barbach (Plume, 1998).

The Ultimate Guide to Anal Sex for Women, Tristan Taormino (Cleis Press, 1998).

Your Sexual Secrets: When to Keep Them, When and How to Tell, Marty Klein (Pacifica Press, 1988).

BOOKS ON TANTRA AND TAOISM

The Art of Everyday Ecstasy: The Seven Tantric Keys for Bringing Passion, Spirit and Joy into Every Part of Your Life, Margo Anand (Broadway Books, 1999).

The Art of Sexual Ecstasy: The Path of Sacred Sexuality for Western Lovers, Margo Anand (Tarcher, 1988).

The Art of Sexual Magic: Cultivating Sexual Energy to Transform Your Life, Margot Anand.

The Complete Kama Sutra: The First Unabridged Modern Translation of the Classic Indian Text, Alain Danielou, trans. (Inner Traditions International Ltd., 1995).

Ecstasy Through Tantra (Llewellyns Tantra and Sexual Arts Series), Jonn Mumford (Llewllyn Publications, 1988).

Healing Love through the Tao: Cultivating Female Sexual Energy, Mantak Chia and Maneewan Chia (Healing Tao Books, 1986).

Sacred Orgasms, Kenneth Ray Stubbs (Secret Garden, 1992).

Sexual Energy Ecstasy: A Practical Guide to Lovemaking Secrets of the East and West, David Ramsdale, et al. (Bantam Doubleday Dell, 1993).

Sexual Secrets: The Alchemy of Ecstasy, Nik Douglas and Penny Slinger (Destiny Books, 1979).

Spiritual Sex: Secrets of Tantra from the Ice Age to the New Millennium, Nik Douglas (Pocket Books, 1997).

The Tao of Love and Sex: The Ancient Chinese Way to Ecstasy, Jolan Chang (Penguin, 1997).

The Tao of Sexual Massage, Stephen Russell (Fireside, 1992).

Taoist Secrets of Love: Cultivating Male Sexual Energy, Mantak Chia and Maneewan Chia (Healing Tao Books, 1986).

The Yin-Yang Butterfly, Valentin Chu (Putnam, 1994).

An exhaustive bibliography of books and Web sites on all aspects of Tantra can be found in *Spiritual Sex* by Nik Douglas. Various Web sites offer a wide selection of books on Taoism.

VIDEOS ON FEMALE SEXUAL RESPONSE

Carol Queen's Great Vibrations: An Explicit Consumer Guide to Vibrators, Carol Queen and Joani Blank (Blank Tapes Productions, 1995).

Celebrating Orgasm: Women's Private Self-loving Sessions, Betty Dodson (Betty Dodson, 1996).

Faces of Ecstasy, Joani Blank (Blank Tapes Productions, 1995).

Fire in the Valley: An Intimate Guide to Female Genital Massage, Annie Sprinkle and Joseph Kramer (EroSpirit Research Institute, 1999).

How to Female Ejaculate, Fanny Fatale (Blush Entertainment, 1992).

The Magic of Female Ejaculation, Dorrie Lane (House O'Chicks, 1992).

Nice Girls... Films by and about Women (#11 Nice Girls Do It Nice), Kathy Daymond and Shannon Bell (Picture Start, Inc., 1989).

Orgasmic Expulsions of Fluid in the Sexually Stimulated Female, Beverly Whipple (Focus International, 1981).

Self-Loving: A Video Portrait of a Women's Sexuality Seminar, Betty Dodson (Betty Dodson, 1991).

Sluts and Goddesses, Maria Beatty and Annie Sprinkle (Beatty/ Sprinkle, 1992).

Viva la Vulva: Women's Sex Organs Revealed, Betty Dodson (Betty Dodson, 1998).

Women Who Love Sex: Creating New Images of Our Sexual Selves—A Video Conversation with Gina Ogden and Others, Gina Ogden (Gina Ogden, 1999). www.womanspirit.net

These videos are available through most sexuality boutiques and some video stores, as well as through online catalogs and bookstores.

SEXUALITY RESOURCES ON THE WORLD WIDE WEB
Sexuality Information, Education, Points of View, Works of Art and Workshops

http://www.susiebright.com: Susie Bright presents a no-glitz, no-nonsense, serious Web site dedicated to "first-rate reading material." The site includes intriguing essays and interviews, excerpts from cutting-edge books and Susie Sexpert's own columns, including her famous Dan Quayle wet dream. Bright aficionados can pick up current riffs from playboy.com.

http://www.gatesofheck.com: Annie Sprinkle's site provides news on sexual politics and a selection of her favorite tomes on sex, as well as her own intellectually provocative books and videos. The gallery contains her famous "bosom ballet," her equally well-known "public cervix announcement" including information on how to do vaginal and cervical self-examination, plus her unique "tit prints" for purchase. There is also a rich collection of links to sites of Annie's friends, pages devoted to spiritual sexuality, online sexzines, and sexual politics sites.

http://www.bettydodson.com: Betty Dodson, the godmother of masturbation, has a diverse site featuring information on her groundbreaking videos, her personal sexual memoirs, discussion on every facet of masturbation, a gallery of genital art, a rich list of Q&As, her outspoken opinions on sexual politics and censorship, fantasy, humor, and more.

http://www/bodyelectric.org: The renowned Body Electric School site provides the extensive workshop schedule, faculty bios, massage products, and a host of home study videos.

http://www.hai.org: The Human Awareness Institute offers workshops on sexual intimacy; the site describes the institute's program and provides information on the schedule, instructors, and how to sign up.

http://www.croyalle.com: In this site, Candida Royalle, the former porn star who pioneered women-oriented erotic movies, touts her own erotic films and videos, answers visitors' questions in a lively forum, and offers a catalog of sexy products, including "anatomically correct vibrators" designed especially for women. "Out and About With Candida" chronicles her latest adventures in the erotic universe and "Behind the Scenes" contains her firsthand account of the making of her erotic videos.

http://www.sexuality.org: The Society for Human Sexuality site is a huge online archive that includes advice on many sexuality issues; extensive guides to books, sex toys, erotica and video rentals; information on safer sex practices; erotic massage; and interviews with sexuality educators. It also provides comprehensive links to sexuality sites.

http://www.jackinworld.com: Devoted exclusively to information on masturbation, this site provides how-to tips and information, Q&As, separate chat rooms for adolescents and adults, reader contributions, and a new "masturbation life story" each month. Excellent information for teens and adults.

http://www.condomania.com: The activist entrepreneurs at Condomania offer a voluminous site featuring every imaginable condom and other sexual accoutrements, such as lubricant, for mail-order purchase, as well as clear, accurate information on safer sex, news items, and links to sites dedicated to promoting safer sex, AIDS awareness education, and a positive sexuality.

http://www.sfsi.org: The site of the famous San Francisco Sex Information project provides FAQs (frequently asked questions) and online sexuality advice, therapy referrals, a list of classes, and links to medical information and support groups.

http://www.plannedparenthood.org: The Planned Parenthood Web site offers reliable information on birth control and emergency contraception, sexually transmitted diseases, pregnancy and parenting, abortion, teen issues, and women's health.

http://www.opr.princeton.edu/ec/: Sponsored by the Office of Population Research of Princeton University, this site provides information on emergency contraception (the "morning-after pill"), Q&As, and a national list of providers.

http://www.sexualhealth.com: The site of the Sexual Health Network provides answers to FAQs, as well as information on sexuality and disability, sex over forty, transgender issues, and parenting options. It also provides continuing education and training for health professionals.

http://www.sexed.org: Dr. Marty Klein, a marriage and family counselor for twenty years, teaches human sexuality at the Stanford Medical School, and writes user-friendly books on sexuality. His site features Q&As from *Ask Me Anything: A Sex Therapist Answers the Most Important Question of the 1990s*, and information on his other books such as *Let Me Count the Ways: Discovering Great Sex Without Intercourse*. The site also includes an article archive, a sexuality library, information on books, audio- and videotapes, as well as hot links.

http://www.bluesinthebedroom.com: Dr. Judy Kuransky, a well-known sex therapist, provides advice and tips on sexuality for people taking medication for depression, including "Facts about Clinical Depression," "Sexual Problems: A Symptom of Depression," and "Little Known Facts About Antidepressants."

http://www.sfbg.com/asc: Andrea Nemerson teaches human sexuality and trains phone volunteers at San Francisco Sex Information and runs workshops on sexuality and verbal self-defense skills for community groups. During her tenure at SFSI and through her column for the *San Francisco Bay Guardian*, Andrea has answered thousands of questions on sexuality. Her site features many of the juiciest ones in a no-holds-barred, nonjudgmental manner.

http://www.drruth.com: The famous Dr. Ruth Westheimer provides sex tips and answers visitors' questions for teens, adults, and seniors, as well as a useful listing of books and videos.

http://www.goaskalice.columbia.edu: In this site sponsored by Columbia University, experts answer real questions from real people on such issues as relationships, sexuality, and sexual and emotional health.

http://www.askisadora.com: Nationally syndicated columnist Isadora Alman offers a public forum "for mature discussion of sexuality and relationships." Her own books and tapes garnered from her columns over the years are available for purchase.

http://www.yoursexcoach.com: Well-known activist and sex therapist Dr. Patti Britton personally answers readers' questions and provides an archive of Q&As as well, and in the "Confessional," visitors admit their deepest sexual secrets and desires.

http://www.tantra.com: One of many useful sites devoted to Tantra, including books, videos, music, audiotapes, products, and access to several discussion forums.

http://gloria-brame.com: This site by Gloria G. Brame, coauthor of *Different Loving: The World of Dominance and Submission* and doyenne of S/M aficionados, is billed as "an eclectic literary domain for free-thinkers" and includes pages on literature, politics and technology, kinky sex, relationships, even Tantric sex tips, and "kink links."

http://www.fwhc.org: The official Web site of the Federation of Feminist Women's Health Centers sells *A New View of a Woman's Body* and other books on Women's health.

http://www.progressivehealth.org: Suzann Gage's Progressive Health Services, 8240 Santa Monica Blvd., West Hollywood, CA 90046; phone: 323-650-1508; sells *A New View of a Women's Body*.

Sexuality Boutiques and Catalogs

This list is growing exponentially, and as Mae West once said, "Too much of a good thing can be a good thing." There are enormous similarities in what these catalogs provide, but significant differences too, so each one merits a look. If it's available, it's probably in one of these catalogs. In addition, many of these sites offer lively columns, sex advice by well-known experts, entertainment links, and much more.

Adam and Eve, http://www.adameve.com; phone: 800-274-0333.

Blowfish: Good Products for Great Sex, http://www.blowfish.com.

Come As You Are, http://www.comeasyouare.com; 701 Queen St. West, Toronto, ON, Canada M6J 1E6; phone: 416-504-7934; fax: 416-504-7490.

Eve's Garden, http://www.evesgarden.com; 119 West 57 St., 12th Floor, New York, NY 10019; phone: 800-848-3837 or 212-757-8651; fax: 212-977-4306.

Good Vibrations, http://www.goodvibes.com; 1210 Valencia St., San Francisco, CA 94110; phone: 800-289-8423; fax: 415-974-0980 and 2504 San Pablo Ave. (at Dwight), Berkeley, CA 94702; phone: 510-841-8987.

Grand Opening!, http://www.grandopening.com; 318 Harvard St. #32, Brookline, MA 02446; phone: 617-731-2626; fax: 617-731-2693.

Naiad Press, http://www.naiadpress.com; P.O. Box 10543, Tallahassee, FL 32302; phone: 850-539-5965.

Nice-N-Naughty, http://www.nice-n-naughty.com; Passion Flower, 4 Yosemite Avenue, Oakland, CA 94611; phone: 510-601-7750.

Pleasure Chest, http://www.net101.com/rocknroll/pleasure.html; 7733 Santa Monica Boulevard, West Hollywood, CA 90046; phone: 800-75DILDO or 213-650-1022; fax: 213-650-1176.

Renaissance Discovery International, http://www.sexhealth.org; email: service@sexhealth.org; phone: 514-844-3434; fax: 514-844-3535.

SensualSource, http://www.sensualsource.com.

The Sexuality Library, http://www.goodvibs.com; 938 Howard Street, #101, San Francisco, CA 94103; phone: 800-289-8423; fax: 415-974-8989.

Toys in Babeland, http://www.babeland.com; email: dena@babeland.com; 711 East Pike Street, Seattle, WA 98122; phone: 800-658-9119; and 91 Rivington St., New York, NY 10002; phone: 212-375-1701.

A Woman's Touch, http://www.a-womans-touch.com; 600 Williamson St., Madison, WI 53703; phone: 888-621-8880 or 608-250-1928.

Womyn'sWare, http://www.womynsware.com; 896 Commercial Drive, Vancouver, BC, Canada U5L 3Y5; phone: 888-WYM-WARE (in North America) or 604-254-2543 (outside of North America).

Xandria Collection, http://www.xandria.com;165 Valley Drive, Brisbane, CA 94005, phone: 415-468-3812.

Academic Sites

http://www.rki.de/gesund/archiv/first.htm: Founded by Erwin Haberle, one of the reigning deans of international sexology and funded by the German government, this site is dedicated to promoting, protecting, and preserving sexual health. It offers articles on the history of sexology, papers and reviews on a wide variety of issues, courses in sexology, a worldwide directory of institutes, organizations, resource centers, training programs, and scientific journals devoted to sexuality, as well as a copy of the World Health Organization's report on sexual health. In German, English, and Spanish. Haberle encourages submissions of useful materials.

http://www.iashs.edu: The Institute for the Advanced Study of Human Sexuality, a private institute, offers a variety of academic degree and clinical certification programs. Its Web site contains a complete catalog describing the curricula, staff credentials, the *Electronic Journal of Human Sexuality*, and a description of the library facilities and archives.

http://www.ejhs.org: This site provides direct access to the *Electronic Journal of Human Sexuality*, published by the Institute for the Advanced Study of Human Sexuality.

Advocacy and Professional Sexuality Organizations

http://www.siecus.org: Web site of the Sexuality Information and Education Council of the United States that features information for parents on children's questions about sexuality, a discussion of religion and sexuality ("What the Bible Says About Sexuality," among other topics), a list of publications, a compilation of sexuality laws state by state, guidelines for comprehensive sexuality education, a community action kit, and resources for underserved communities and communities of color.

http://www.aascct.org: The American Association of Sex Educators, Counselors, and Therapists is a professional association that includes physicians, nurses, social workers, psychologists, allied health professionals, clergy, lawyers, sociologists, marriage and family counselors and therapists, family planning specialists and researchers, as well as students in relevant professional disciplines who share an interest in promoting understanding of human sexuality and healthy sexual behavior. The organization provides certification and education of sexuality educators, counselors, and therapists. The site supports the publication and dissemination of professional materials related to these fields.

http://www.plannedparenthood.org: The national Planned Parenthood site covers many bases including abortion, birth control, pregnancy and parenting, and includes current news and articles on reproductive rights, FAQs, and an extensive database on these issues.

http://www.ssc.wisc.edu/ssss/: The Society for the Scientific Study of Sexuality (SSSS or "Quad S") site posts announcements of meetings, conferences, grants, and awards, as well as contents and other information for the society's various publications including its newsletter *Sexual Science*, and *The Journal of Sex Research* and *Annual Review of Sex Research*.

Sites for Teens

A number of informative sex-positive Web sites dedicated to the needs and interests of teens serve about any topic of concern. Parents: Want to know what children think about sexuality and how to answer uncomfortable questions? Check out these sites.

http://www.gurl.com: Among many issues, this comprehensive site for teenage girls and those on the cusp of adolescence is an excellent antidote to parental reluctance or inability to discuss sex, as well as to fear-based government-sponsored "sexuality education" programs. Teens can turn to sites such as this one to find reliable, nonjudgmental information on sexuality by experts and teens themselves and a secure place to chat and ask questions.

http://www.itsyoursexlife.com: Jointly sponsored by MTV and the Kaiser Family Foundation, this teen-oriented site features current news about sexuality, information on pregnancy and contraception, STDs, and sexual communication.

http://www.flash.net/~nmtpc: The New Mexico Teen Pregnancy Coalition provides information on pregnancy prevention, parenting, male involvement, and the rights of teen parents in school.

http://www.teenwire.com: This lively site devoted to sexual health includes news, articles, quizzes, answers to "real questions from teens," a teen zine and profiles of teens who are standing up, speaking out, and taking action on a variety of issues.

For more extensive listings on Web sites on every topic, see *The Woman's Guide to Sex on the Web*, by Anne Semans and Cathy Winks (HarperSanFrancisco, 1999) and *The Joy of Cybersex: A Guide for Creative Lovers* by Deb Levine, two useful and reliable guides to sexuality sites on the World Wide Web.

REFERENCES

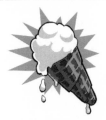

1 Kinsey, Alfred, et al., *Sexual Behavior of the Human Female*. Philadelphia: W.B. Saunders, 1953, 626-627.

2 Tavris, Carol, *The Mismeasure of Woman: Why Women Are Not the Better Sex, the Inferior Sex, or the Opposite Sex*. New York: Simon & Schuster/Touchstone, 1992, 244.

3 Frank, Anne, *The Diary of Anne Frank: The Definitive Edition*. New York: Bantam Books, 1997, 235-236.

4 Mayer, Ruth, "MISH," from "New Framework for Fear-Based, Abstinence-only Education." The SIECUS Report, 25:4, 14-17.

5 Downer, Carol, personal communication.

6 Sherfey, Mary Jane, *The Nature and Evolution of Female Sexuality*. New York: Random House, 1972.

7 Federation of Feminist Women's Health Centers, *A New View of a Woman's Body: An Illustrated Guide*, Tenth anniversary ed., Los Angeles: Feminist Health Press, 1991.

8 Dodson, Betty, "Viva la Vulva: Women's Sex Organs Revealed." Betty Dodson, 1998.

9 Downer, Carol, personal communication.

10 Komisaruk, Barry R. and Beverly Whipple, "Physiological and perceptual correlates of orgasm produced by genital and non-genital stimulation." *Proceedings of the First International Conference on Orgasm*, Bombay: VRP Publishers, 1991, 69-72.

11 Fell, Alison, in *Straight Sex: Rethinking the Politics of Pleasure,* Lynne Segal, ed. Berkeley: University of California Press, 1994, 39-40.

12 Schwartz, Kit, *The Female Member.* New York: St. Martin's Press, 1988.

13 Laqueur, Thomas, *Making Sex: The Body and Gender From the Greeks to Freud.* Cambridge: Harvard University Press, 1990, vii.

14 Galen, Claudius, *On the Usefulness of the Parts of the Body XIV.6.* Margaret T. May, trans. Ithaca: Cornell University Press, 1968. Quoted in Laqueur, 26.

15 Laqueur, 70.

16 Estienne, Charles, *La Dissection des parti du corpus humain,* 1546. Quoted in Laqueur, 133.

17 Laqueur, 64-65.

18 Sharp, Jane, *The Midwives Book, or the Whole Art of Midwifery Discovered Directing Childbearing Women How to Behave Themselves in their Conception, Breeding, Bearing and Nursing Children.* London, 1671. Quoted in Laqueur, 65.

19 Laqueur, 149.

20 Laqueur, 157.

21 Voltaire, "Women," in *Philosophical Dictionary,* quoted in "A Sampling of Eighteenth Century Philosophy," from *A History of Women: Renaissance and Enlightenment Paradoxes,* Natalie Zemon Davis and Arlette Farge, eds. Cambridge: Belknap/Harvard, 1993, 326.

22 Rousseau, Jean Jacques, *Emile.* New York: Everyman's Library, 1993

23 Crampe-Casnabet, Michele, *A History of Women: Renaissance and Enlightenment Paradoxes,* ed. by Natalie Zemon Davis and Arlette Farge, Cambridge: Belknap/Harvard, 1993.

24 Acton, William, *The Function and Disorders of the Reproductive Organs in Childhood, Youth, Adult Age, and Advanced Life, Considered in their Physiological, Social and Moral Relations,* 1857. Quoted in Laqueur, 196.

25 Kobelt, George Ludwig, "The Female Sex Organs in Humans and Some Mammals." In *The Classic Clitoris,* Thomas P. Lowry, ed. Chicago: Nelson Hall, 1978, 19-55.

26 Freud, Sigmund, *Three Essays on the Theory of Sexuality* in *Freud on Women: A Reader*, Elisabeth Bruehl, ed. New York: Norton, 1990, 137.

27 Laqueur, 157.

28 Moore, Lisa Jean and Adele E. Clarke, "Clitoral Conventions and Transgressions: Graphic Representations in Anatomy Texts, c1900-1991." *Feminist Studies* 21:2, Summer 1995, 255-301.

29 Dickinson, Robert Latou, *Human Sex Anatomy: A Topographical Hand Atlas.* Baltimore: Williams and Wilkinson, 1949.

30 Thomas, C. L., ed., *Taber's Cyclopedic Medical Dictionary.* New York: Eliot Books, 1981, 581.

31 Masters, William H. and Virginia E. Johnson, *Human Sexual Response.* New York: Little, Brown, 1966, 45.

32 Sherfey, Mary Jane, *The Nature and Evolution of Female Sexuality*, New York: Random House, 1972, 112.

33 Whipple, Beverly, personal communication.

34 Walsh, Patrick C., et al., eds., *Campbell's Urology*, Sixth ed., Philadelphia: W. B. Saunders Company, 1986, 233-274.

35 Ladas, Alice Kahn, Beverly Whipple, and John Perry, *The G Spot and Other Discoveries about Human Sexuality.* Holt, Rinehart and Winston, 1982.

36 Sevely, Josephine Lowndes and J. W. Bennett, "Concerning Female Ejaculation and the Female Prostate." *Journal of Sex Research* 14, 1-20.

37 Sevely, Josephine Lowndes, *Eve's Secrets: A New Theory of Female Sexuality.* New York: Random House, 1987, 47-48.

38 Perry, J. D. and Whipple, B., "Pelvic Muscle Strength of Female Ejaculators: Evidence to Support a New Theory of Orgasm." *Journal of Sex Research,* 1981, 17(1).

39 Ladas, Whipple, and Perry, 76.

40 Ibid.

41 Belzer, Edwin G., "Orgasmic Expulsions of Women: A Review and Heuristic Inquiry." *Journal of Sex Research 17,* 1-12.

42 Cabello Santamaria, F. and R. Nesters, "Female Ejaculation: Myths and Reality." Paper given at the 13th Congress of Sexology, Barcelona, Spain, August 29, 1997.

43 Sevely, 92.

44 Ladas, Whipple, and Perry, 69.

45 Heath, Desmond, "An Investigation into the Origins of a Copious Vaginal Discharge During Intercourse: Enough to Wet the Bed—That Is Not Urine." *Journal of Sex Research* 20:2, May 1984, 197.

46 Sevely, 93.

47 Ladas, Whipple, and Perry, 68.

48 Sellavy, E. Rose, "Shooting Ain't Just for the Boys!" *The Urban Herbalist,* No. 9, July 1993.

49 Whipple, Beverly, personal communication.

50 Kinsey, Alfred, et al., *Sexual Behavior in the Human Female.* Philadelphia: W. B. Saunders, 1953, 612.

51 Masters, William M., Virginia E. Johnson, with Robert C. Kolodny, *Masters and Johnson on Sex and Human Loving.* Boston: Little, Brown and Company, 1986, 79–80.

52 Heath, 196.

53 Fatale, Fanny, *On Our Backs,* Sept. 1992, 8.

54 Tiefer, Leonore, personal communication.

55 Everett, Houston, "The Detailed Anatomy of the Paraurethral Ducts in the Adult Human Female." *American Journal of Obstetrics and Gynecology* 55, 1948, 101.

56 Gittes, Ruben L., personal communication.

57 Douglas, Nik and Penny Slinger, *Sexual Secrets: The Alchemy of Ecstasy.* Rochester, VT: Destiny Books, 1979, 278-279.

58 *The Kama Sutra of Vatsyayana,* Richard Burton, trans. New York: Putnam, 1966, 186.

59 Quoted in Fantham, E., et al., *Women in the Classical World.* New York: Oxford University Press, p. 186.

60 Quoted in Laqueur, 33.

61 Quoted in Laqueur, 40.

62 Quoted in Laqueur, 64.

63 Quoted in Laqueur, 92-93.

64 de Graaf, Regnier, "New Treatise Concerning the Generative Organs of Women." *Journal of Reproduction and Fertility*, supp. no. 17, 77-222.

65 Skene, Alexander, "The Anatomy and pathology of two important glands of the female urethra." *American Journal of Obstetrics and Diseases of Women and Children* 13, 265-270.

66 Netter, Frank H., *The CIBA Collection of Medical Illustrations, Volume 2: A Compilation of Paintings on the Normal and Pathologic Anatomy of the Reproductive System*. CIBA, 1954, 106.

67 Van de Velde, Theodore H., *Ideal Marriage: Its Physiology and Technique*. New York: Random House, 1957, 195-96.

68 Huffman, J. W., "The Detailed Anatomy of the Paraurethral Ducts in the Adult Human Female." *American Journal of Obstetrics and Gynecology* 55, 1948, 86-101.

69 Grafenberg, Ernest, "The Role of the Urethra in Female Orgasm." *International Journal of Sexology* 3, 1950, 147.

70 Sevely, Josephine Lowndes, *Eve's Secrets: A New Theory of Female Sexuality*. New York: Random House, 1987.

71 Whipple, Beverly, personal communication.

72 Ladas, Whipple, and Perry.

73 Whipple, Beverly, personal communication.

74 O'Connell, Helen E., et al., "Anatomical Relationship Between Urethra and Clitoris." *Journal of Urology* 159, 1892.

75 Michael, R. T. et al., *Sex in America: A Definitive Survey*, New York: Little, Brown and Company, 1994, 135.

76 Francoeur, Robert T., et al., 575.

77 Christina, Greta, "Are We Having Sex Now or What?" in *The Erotic Impulse*, David Steinberg, ed. Tarcher, 1992, 24-29.

78 Kinsey, Alfred, et al., 142

79 Whipple, Beverly, William E. Hartman, and Marilyn Fithian, "Orgasm," in *Human Sexuality: An Encyclopedia*, Vernon L. Bullough and Bonnie Bullough, eds. New York: Garland Publishing, Inc., 1994, 430-433.

80 Whipple, Beverly, personal communication.

81 Bogus, Sdiane, "Dyke Hands," in *Erotique Noire/Black Erotica*, M. Decosta-Willis, R. Martin and R. P. Bell, eds. New York: Doubleday, 1992, 198-199

82 Giorgi, G. and M. Siccardi, "Ultrasonigraphic Observation of the Female Fetus' Sexual Behavior in Utero," letter in the *American Journal of Obstetrics and Gynecology* 175, Sept. 1996, 753.

83 Tannahill, Reay, *Sex in History*. New York: Stein and Day, 1980, 342.

84 Lissarrague, Francois, "The Sexual Life of Satyrs," in *Before Sexuality: The Construction of Erotic Experience in the Ancient Greek World*, David M. Halperin, John J. Winkler, and Froma I. Zeitlin, eds. Princeton: Princeton University Press, 1990, 57.

85 Maines, Rachel P., *The Technology of Orgasm: "Hysteria," the Vibrator, and Women's Sexual Satisfaction*. Baltimore: Johns Hopkins University Press, 1999, 23.

86 Jacquart, Danielle and Claude Thomasset, *Sexuality and Medicine in the Middle Ages*. Princeton: Princeton University Press, 1988, 147-155.

87 Genesis 39:9, *The New Annotated Bible*,. New York: Oxford University Press, 1991, 49-50.

88 Tissot, S.A.A.D., *Onanism: A Treatise on the Diseases Produced by Masturbation, Or, the Dangerous Effects of Secret and Excessive Venery*. A. Hume, trans. London: J. Pridden, 1761.

89 Greico, Sara F. Matthews, "The Body, Appearance, and Sexuality," in *A History of Women: III. Renaissance and Enlightenment Paradoxes*, Georges Duby and Michelle Perrot, eds. Cambridge: Harvard University Press, 1993, 72.

90 Wollstonecraft, Mary, *Thoughts on the Education of Daughters*. London, 1787, 82. Quoted in Laqueur, 203.

91 Nissenbaum, Stephen, *Sex, Diet and Debility in Jacksonian America: Sylvester Graham and Health Reform*. Westport, CT, 1980, 30, 110.

92 Michael, et al., 161.

93 Kinsey, et al., 142.

94 Dodson, Betty, *Sex for One: The Joy of Selfloving.* New York: Crown, 1987.

95 Barbach, Lonnie Garfield, *For Yourself: The Fulfillment of Female Sexuality.* New York: Doubleday, 1976.

96 Hite, Shere, *The Hite Report: A Nationwide Study of Female Sexuality.* New York: Dell Publishing Co., 1976.

97 Tiefer, Leonore, "The Right Wing Attack on Sexuality: The Backlash Against Masturbation." Paper delivered to The American Public Health Association, November 11, 1996.

98 Quoted in Cole, W., and L. Phillips, *Sex: The Most Fun You Can Have Without Laughing and Other Quotations.* New York: St. Martin's Press, 1990, 101.

99 Fatout, Paul, ed., *Mark Twain Speaking.* Iowa City: University of Iowa Press, 1976, 125.

100 Winks, Cathy and Anne Semans, *The Good Vibrations Guide to Sex.* Philadelphia and San Francisco: Cleis Press, 1994, 57-58.

101 Francoeur, R. T., eds., *The Complete Dictionary of Sexology.* New York: Continuum, 1995, 381.

102 Maines, 104.

103 Dodson, Betty, personal communication.

104 Blank, J., *Good Vibrations: The Complete Guide to Vibrators.* San Francisco: Down There Press, 1989.

105 Taylor, Timothy, *The Prehistory of Sex: Four Million Years of Human Sexual Culture.* New York: Bantam Books, 1997, 177, 129.

106 Winks and Semans, p. 156.

107 Queen, Carol A., "Sisters are Doin' It For Themselves," *On Our Backs*, November/December, 1992, 22.

108 Rifaat, Alifa, "My World of the Unknown," in *The Penguin Book of Erotic Stories by Women*, R. G. Jones, and A. S. Williams, eds. New York: Viking, 1995, 207-221.

109 Friday, Nancy, *Women on Top: How Real Life Has Changed Women's Sexual Fantasies.* New York: Pocket Books, 1991.

Estienne, Charles, 78, 242
Eve's Garden, 185, 235
exhibitionism, 109, 199-200, 224
Fallopian tubes, 79, 200
    See also egg tubes.
Fallopius, Gabriel, 78
family planning, 135, 238
fantasies, 18, 22, 53, 136, 143, 153, 158-161,
    164, 166-167, 174, 200, 215, 217, 220, 247
fasting, 143
Fatale, Fanny, 109, 113, 228, 244
Federation of Feminist Women's Health Centers
    (FFWHCs), 9, 11-15, 17, 31, 34-35, 37, 40,
    46, 54, 73, 89-90, 95-96, 105, 217, 234, 241
Fell, Alison, 68, 241
female ejaculation, 17-18, 23, 43, 91-93, 95-97,
    100, 102-114, 116-120, 122, 124-126, 192-
    193, 200, 228, 243
female genital mutilation, 60
female prostate, 54, 93, 114-117, 121-124, 126,
    200, 206, 243
female sexual response, 228
female sexuality, 9, 17, 34, 91, 95, 124, 146,
    170, 215-217, 224, 241, 243, 245-247
feminism, 11, 215
feminists, 13-14, 16-18, 31, 60, 71, 89, 92, 126,
    129-130, 134, 144, 151
fetus, 93, 118, 139, 246
FFWHCs. *See* Federation of Feminist Women's
    Health Centers
fidelity, 142
Focus on the Family, 28
foreplay, 27
foreskin, 32, 36-37, 67, 78, 145, 202

fork, 39, 46, 54, 201, 210
fourchette, 38-39, 54, 201
    See also fork.
Frank, Anne, 24, 26-27, 37, 64, 241
French Revolution, 79
frenulum, 37-38, 54, 197, 201
    See also bridle.
Freud, Sigmund, 74, 82-84, 216, 242
Friday, Nancy, 160, 215, 217, 220, 247
front commissure, 35, 38, 54, 201
fructose, 99
G spot, 43, 94-96, 99, 103, 109, 115, 124-125,
    152, 177, 224, 243
Galen, Claudius, 76, 78, 119, 121-122, 242
gay men, 23, 148, 156, 175
gender identity, 62
gender orientation, 29
gender reassignment surgery, 62
genitals, 21-22, 24, 26-28, 30, 37, 40, 48, 53, 58,
    60, 62, 64, 66-67, 71-72, 74, 76-78, 82, 84,
    86-87, 142, 145, 148, 170, 175, 183, 188-
    190, 201, 204, 207, 210
    mutilation of, 60-61
    self-examination of, 188-189
Gittes, Ruben, 116, 244
glans, 14, 16, 30, 32-34, 36-39, 42, 44-45, 47-
    49, 52-54, 57, 60-61, 65-67, 82-83, 86, 145,
    152, 154, 175, 183, 197, 201-202, 207-210
glucose, 97
Good Vibrations, 147, 149, 152, 193, 224-225,
    235, 247
Grafenberg, Ernest, 123, 245
Grafenberg spot, 94-96
    See also G spot.